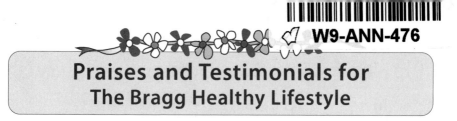

Praises and Testimonials for
The Bragg Healthy Lifestyle

These are just a few of the thousands of testimonials we receive yearly, praising The Bragg Health Books for the rejuvenation benefits they reap – physically, mentally and spiritually. We look forward to hearing from you also.

Thanks to Bragg Health Books, they were our introduction to healthy living. We are very grateful to you and your father.
– Marilyn Diamond, co-author, *Fit For Life*
– Best Seller for 40 weeks

When I was a young Stanford University gymnastics coach Paul Bragg's words and example inspired me to live a healthy lifestyle. I was twenty-three then; now I'm over sixty-two, and my own health and fitness serves as a living testimonial to Bragg's wisdom, carried on by Patricia, his dedicated Health Crusading daughter.
– Dan Millman, author, *Way of the Peaceful Warrior*
www.peacefulwarrior.com

Thanks to the Bragg Fasting Book and the Healthy Lifestyle, we are healthy, fit and singing better and staying younger than ever!
– The Beach Boys • *www.TheBeachBoys.com*

Thank you Paul and Patricia Bragg for my simple, easy to follow Healthy Lifestyle. You make my days healthy!
– Clint Eastwood, Academy Award Winning Film Producer, Director, Actor and Bragg follower for over 60 years

---

The Bragg Healthy Lifestyle with Fasting has changed my life! I lost weight and my energy levels went through the roof. I look forward to my fasting days. I think better and am a better husband and father. Thank you Patricia, this has been a great blessing in my life. Also, we enjoyed your important health sharing at our "AOL" Conference.
– Byron H. Elton, former VP Entertainment, Time Warner AOL

I give thanks to Paul C. Bragg and his daughter Patricia for their long years of devoted service spreading health and fitness worldwide. It has made a difference in my life and millions of others. – Pat Robertson, Host "700 Club"

Paul Bragg saved my life at 15 when I attended the Bragg Health Crusade in Oakland. I thank Bragg Healthy Lifestyle for my long, healthy, active life spreading health and fitness. – Jack LaLanne, Thankful Bragg follower to 96^{1}/$_{2}$ years

As a youth I had a learning disability and was told I would never read, write or communicate normally. At 14 I dropped out of school and at 17 ended up in Hawaii surfing. My road to recovery led me to Paul Bragg who changed my life by giving me one simple affirmation: "I am a genius and I apply my wisdom." Bragg inspired me to go back to school and get my education and from there miracles happened. I have authored 72 training programs and 40 books and love to crusade around the world thanks to Paul Bragg. – Dr. John Demartini, Dynamic Crusader Star in "The Secret" • www.DrDemartini.com

I regained my health by eating organic foods and vegetables and taking supplements. I'm eating foods the way God created them and my body is thriving. Thanks for Bragg Healthy Lifestyle – it's great! – Candace Hawthorne, Metairie, LA

Your dad, Dr. Paul C. Bragg IS the FATHER of the Natural Health Industry and the entire Natural Health Movement. Everything that has been done in Natural Health and Physical Culture since has been based on the dedicated pioneering vision and principles articulated by Dr. Paul C. Bragg. He gave us all our strong direction! – Dr. William Wong, TX

Your father Paul Bragg was a great man and he brought health and nutrition into our world! – Julia Childs, American Chef

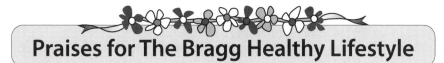

Praises for The Bragg Healthy Lifestyle

Bragg Books were my conversion to the healthy way.
– James F. Balch, M.D.,
co-author, *Prescription for Nutritional Healing*

The Bragg Healthy Lifestyle teaches you to take control of your health and build a healthy, fulfilled, long life.
– Mark Victor Hansen, co-producer,
Chicken Soup for Soul Series

I'm a champion weight lifter at Muscle Beach (50 years) and I am a big Bragg fan. – Chris Baioa, Santa Monica, CA

I met Paul Bragg in 1964 at "L" Street Beach in Boston. Both Paul and his daughter Patricia are dynamic, energetic and life-changers! They have always been health inspirations to millions around the world, but especially to me! I gave my first lecture with them in April 1964, I was 22, I am over 64 now. Patricia has more energy than any 3 people I know put together and loves traveling the world for Bragg Health Crusades.
– Dr. David Carmos and Dr. Shawn Miller,
co-authors of *You're Never Too Old To Become Young*

Warm wishes all the way from Malaysia to express my sincere gratitude to both of you for sharing your wonderful secret of youth through the Bragg Healthy Lifestyle Living. – Marlyn Lim, Sarawak, Malaysia

---

I had the opportunity to sit next to Patricia on a flight from Dallas to Los Angeles. Her honesty about my weight and health really inspired me to make a life change. One year later, I am 85 lbs. lighter and heart rate cut almost in half.
Patricia you helped save my life! – Mike Ableman, TX

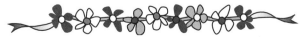

Kindness should be a frame of mind in which we are alert to every chance: to do, to give, to share and to cheer. – Patricia Bragg

Thank you Patricia for our first meeting in London in 1968. You gave me your *The Miracle of Fasting* Book, it got me exercising, brisk walking and eating more wisely. You were a blessing God-sent.
– Reverend Billy Graham

In 1975 I was diagnosed with coronary heart disease. I followed the Free Bragg Exercise Classes and Lectures at Fort DeRussy in Waikiki, six times a week. Over 31 years have passed and am now 84-years young thanks to Bragg Healthy Lifestyle. – Helen Risk, RN, Hawaii

---

It was in Hawaii I began to realize that while lifestyle choices can not only be a major negative to health and well-being, but lifestyle can be a winning asset to wellness! My discovery on fitness and health began shortly after I arrived in Hawaii at 19 when I discovered fitness and health pioneer Paul Bragg teaching a free exercise class 6 days a week at Waikiki Beach. Bragg inspired my future.
– Kathy Smith, Hollywood, CA • *www.KathySmith.com*
Kathy has sold millions of fitness videos, more than anyone!

Patricia, it was such an honor to meet you well over 15 years ago, before I was aware of the fabulous Bragg Health Crusades. Now I have been truly blessed by a more in-depth conversation with you about your life as the daughter of Paul C. Bragg and Bragg's amazing history. Thank you for all your knowledge of health and sharing it with the world. We are healthier and happier because of you!!
– With warm regards, Missy Woodward • *www.pcrm.org*
Physician Committee for Responsible Medicine

Thanks for what you and your dad did for the health of people. Forty years ago doctors didn't believe that food had anything to do with your health. Look where we are today. Your dad must be looking down from Heaven seeing huge footprints he made on life of millions of people. God Bless. – Sharon

D

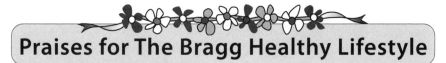

Praises for The Bragg Healthy Lifestyle

Patricia Bragg is a dedicated Health Crusader and she shared her Bragg Healthy Lifestyle with millions of our radio listeners. Thank you Patricia.
– Host George Noory, *Coast to Coast Radio*

How I beat obesity, diabetes, strep and three herniated disks and excruciating pain? The answer was changing to Bragg's Healthy Lifestyle Program! It changed and saved my life! I recovered and also lost over 70 lbs. I received a new life and that is just the beginning because my manhood returned that was lost to diabetes – now that's exciting! On my trip to Honolulu, Hawaii I visited the famous free Bragg Exercise Class at Waikiki Beach. I became so regenerated and happy with new energy that I want the world to join The Bragg Health Crusade. I am deeply thankful to Health Crusaders, Paul and Patricia for my well-being. – Len, Hawaii

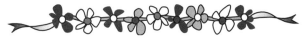

We get letters daily at our Santa Barbara Headquarters. We would love to receive a testimonial from you on any blessings, healings and changes that you have experienced after following The Bragg Healthy Lifestyle and The Miracle of Fasting. It's all within your grasp to be in top health. By following this book, you can reap Super Health and a happy, long, fulfilled life! It's never too late to begin. Read the study (page 97) they did with people in their 80s and 90s and the amazing results that were obtained! Receive miracles with natural nutrition, exercise and some fasting! Start now!

Daily our prayers & love go out to you, your heart, mind & soul. With Love,

| 3 John 2 | *Patricia Bragg* | Genesis 6:3 |

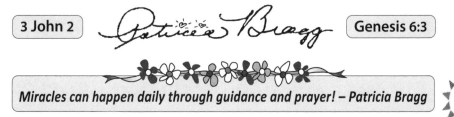

Miracles can happen daily through guidance and prayer! – Patricia Bragg

E

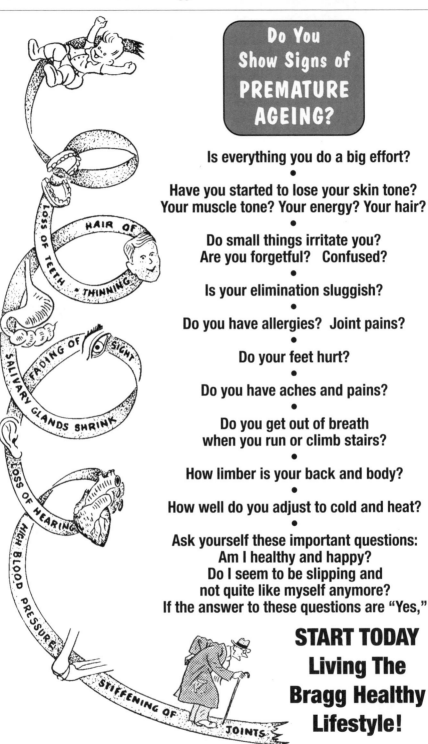

Do You Show Signs of PREMATURE AGEING?

Is everything you do a big effort?

•

Have you started to lose your skin tone?
Your muscle tone? Your energy? Your hair?

•

Do small things irritate you?
Are you forgetful? Confused?

•

Is your elimination sluggish?

•

Do you have allergies? Joint pains?

•

Do your feet hurt?

•

Do you have aches and pains?

•

Do you get out of breath
when you run or climb stairs?

•

How limber is your back and body?

•

How well do you adjust to cold and heat?

•

Ask yourself these important questions:
Am I healthy and happy?
Do I seem to be slipping and
not quite like myself anymore?
If the answer to these questions are "Yes,"

START TODAY Living The Bragg Healthy Lifestyle!

F

He who understands and follows Mother Nature walks with God.

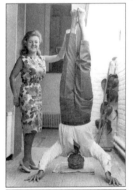

BRAGG PHOTO GALLERY

PATRICIA & PAUL C. BRAGG, N.D., Ph.D.
Dynamic Daughter & Father are World Health Crusaders

BRAGG PRODUCTS
HEALTH IS HERE

During the past century, Bragg Live Food Products developed and pioneered the very first line of Health Foods, from vitamins and minerals to organic nuts, seeds, and sun-dried fruits. This included over 365 health products, – *"one for each day of the year!"* says daughter Patricia Bragg.

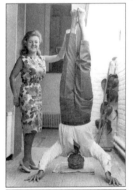

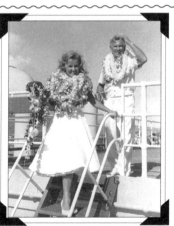

"Thanks for The Bragg Healthy Lifestyle that you shared with me and you are sharing with millions of others worldwide."
– John Gray, Ph.D., author

Picture from
People Magazine August, 1975.

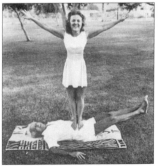

Patricia and father, Paul on world trip in 1950's, during stop in Tahiti.

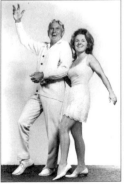

"You have recharged me with joy, hope, love and encouragement, which poured from your words. I am now fasting and using ACV. You have certainly improved my life!"
– Marie Furia, New Jersey

Patricia Bragg stands on her father's stomach. Paul's stomach muscles are so strong he can lift Patricia up and down!

G

PAUL C. BRAGG, N.D., Ph.D.
HEALTH CRUSADER

Life Extension Specialist and Originator of Health Food Stores

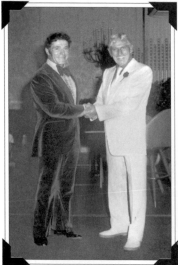

I have experienced a beautiful, remarkable, spiritual and physical awakening since reading Bragg Health Books. I'll never be the same again.
– Sandy Tuttle, Ohio

With every new day comes new strength and new thoughts.
– Eleanor Roosevelt

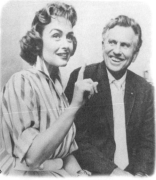

Actress Donna Reed saying "Health First" with Paul C. Bragg.

Dr. Paul C. Bragg (right) Creator Health Food Stores, Pioneer Life Extension Specialist, with his prize student Jack LaLanne. Paul started him on the royal road to health over 85 years ago!

Paul C. Bragg spent much of his time at the Hollywood Studios meeting with top Stars and motion picture industry executives, giving health lectures and private consultations. Dr. Paul C. Bragg was Hollywood's first highly respected, health, fitness and nutrition advisor to the Stars.

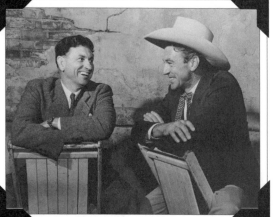

Paul C. Bragg with Gary Cooper, famous American film actor, best known for his many Western films.

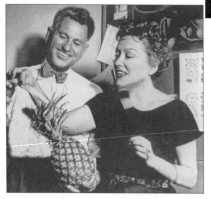

Paul C. Bragg with the famous Hollywood Actress Gloria Swanson, who was leading star in 20s, 30s and 40s. Gloria became a Bragg Health Devotee at 18 and she often would Health Crusade with Bragg during the 1950s.

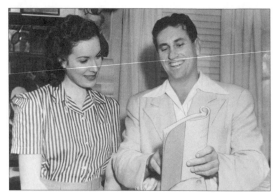

Maureen O'Hara and Paul C. Bragg. This Irish film actress and singer was best noted for playing in "Miracle on 34th Street" and "The Quiet Man."

PAUL C. BRAGG, N.D., Ph.D.
STAYING HEALTHY & FIT

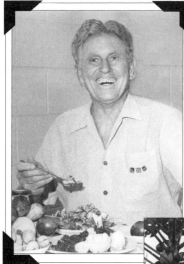

I'd like to thank you for teaching me how to take control of my health! I lost 55 pounds and I feel "great!" Bragg books have showed me vitality, happiness and being close to Mother Nature. You both are real "Crusaders for Health for the World." Thanks!
– Leonard Amato

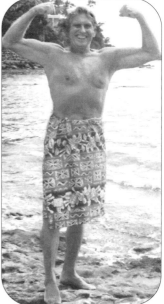

Dr. Paul C. Bragg and daughter Patricia were my early guiding inspiration to my health career.
– Jeffery Bland, Ph.D., Famous Food Scientist

The best thing about the future is that it only comes one day at a time.
– Abraham Lincoln

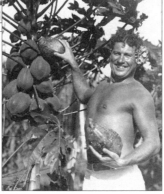

Paul C. Bragg in Tahiti 1920's gathering tropical papaya fruit.

Paul C. Bragg owes his powerful body and superb health to living exclusively on live, vital, healthy, organic rich foods.

Dear Friends – you cannot know how greatly you have impacted my life and some of my friends! We love your Bragg Health Books, teachings and products and are now living healthier, happier lives. Thanks!
– Winnie Brown, Arizona

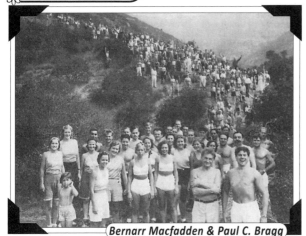

Bernarr Macfadden & Paul C. Bragg

A thousand happy Bragg Health Students enjoy hiking, exercise and fresh air on the trail to Mount Hollywood (above Griffith Observatory) in beautiful California, summer of 1932.

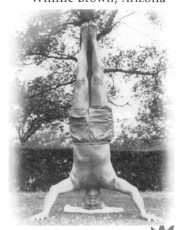

Paul C. Bragg exercising Regent's Park, London.

I

PHOTO GALLERY   PAUL & PATRICIA BRAGG

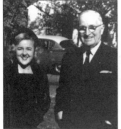

Patricia with 33rd President Harry S. Truman at his home in Independence, Missouri.

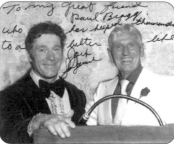

Paul C. Bragg, Creator of Health Food Stores, with his prize student Jack LaLanne, who thanks Bragg for saving his life at 15.

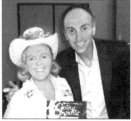

Patrica Bragg with Dr. Jeffrey Smith. He is leader in getting GMO's out of US foods. See GMO video by Jeffrey Smith and narrated by Lisa Oz (Dr. Oz's wife) on web: *GeneticRouletteMovie.com*

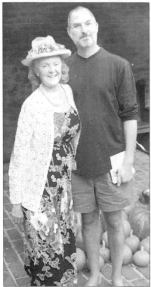

Patricia visiting with Steve Jobs at his home in Palo Alto during the Thanksgiving Holidays.

"I've been reading Bragg Books since high school. I'm thankful for the Bragg Healthy Lifestyle and admire their Health Crusading for a healthier, happier world."
– Steve Jobs, Creator – Apple Computer

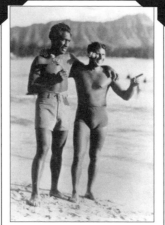

Paul in 1920 with his swimming & surfing friend, Duke Kahanamoku, Waikiki Beach, Diamond Head.

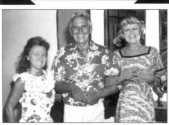

Patricia, Paul C. Bragg and Mrs. Duke (Nadine) Kahanamoku. (Nadine is Patricia's Godmother).

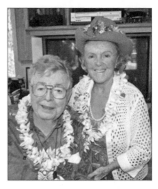

Dr. Earl Bakken with Patricia. He's famous for inventing the first Transistor Pacemaker. His firm Medtronic, developed it and a Resuscitator for fixing ailing hearts that have and are saving thousands of lives. Dr. Bakken lived in Hawaii.

*"I cannot remember a time when the Golden Rule * was not my motto and precept, the torch that guided my footsteps."* – J.C. Penney

*The Golden Rule: Do unto others as you would have them do unto you.

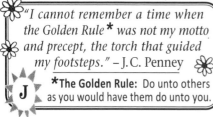

J.C. Penney & Patricia → exercising. They walked often in Palm Springs when he and his wife visited in the winter to enjoy the warm desert sunshine.

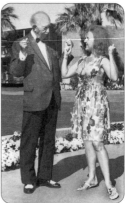

HEALTH CRUSADING TO HOLLYWOOD STARS

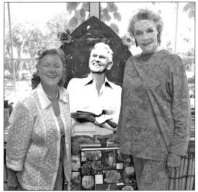

Patricia with friend Actress Jane Russell. Famous Hollywood Star of 40s to 60s.

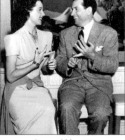

Jane Wyatt learning about health with Paul C. Bragg.

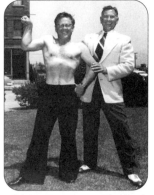

Mickey Rooney with Paul. Rooney was an American film actor and entertainer. He won multiple awards and had one of the longest careers of any actor to age 93!

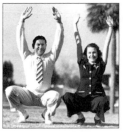

Paul C. Bragg exercising with Actress Helen Parrish.

"Thank you Paul & Patricia Bragg for my simple, easy-to-follow Healthy Lifestyle. You make my days healthy!" – Clint Eastwood, Academy Award Winning Film Producer, Director, Actor and Bragg follower for over 65 years.

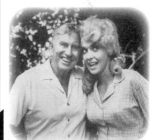

Paul C. Bragg and Donna Douglas, one of Hollywood's most beautiful and talented health advocates. She played the part of "Elly-May" in the *Beverly Hillbillies*, which became one of the longest-running series in television history and was the #1 show in America in its first 2 years.

> **Life is a Miracle Minute by Minute Year by Year!**

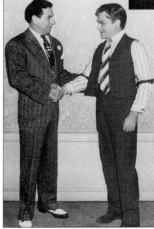

Paul C. Bragg with James Cagney, American film actor. He won major awards for wide variety of roles. The American Film Institute ranked Cagney 8th among the Greatest Male Hollywood Stars of All Time.

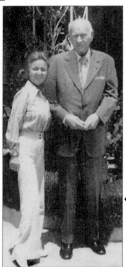

Patricia with Conrad Hilton

← Hotel founder, Conrad Hilton with Patricia Bragg, his Healthy Lifestyle Teacher. *"I wouldn't be alive today if it wasn't for the Braggs and their Bragg Healthy Lifestyle!"* – Conrad Hilton

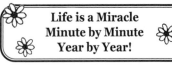

"Thank you for your website. What a wealth of info to learn about how to live and eat healthy. Many Blessings!" – Michel & Mary, California

K

PAUL C. BRAGG, N.D., Ph.D.
PROMOTES HEALTH & FITNESS!

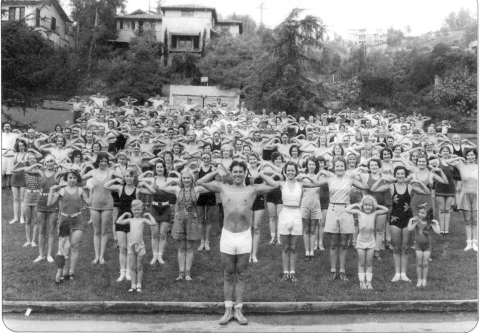

Paul C. Bragg leading an exercise class in Griffith Park, Hollywood, CA – circa 1920s.

Bragg Healthy Lifestyle works Miracles! – Jack LaLanne

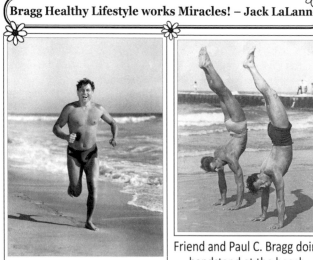

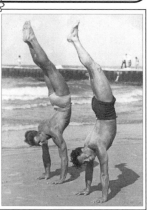

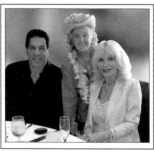

Patricia with Lou and wife Carla at Elaine LaLanne's 90th Birthday Party.

Friend and Paul C. Bragg doing handstand at the beach.

Paul running on Coney Island, New York, where he was a member of the Coney Island Polar Bear Club, known for Cold Water Swimming, 1930s.

TV Hulk Actor Lou Ferrigno gives thanks to Bragg Books. Lou went from puny to become Super Hulk! ➡

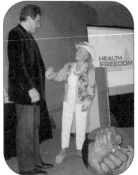

"I lost 102 lbs. with The Bragg Healthy Lifestyle and I have kept it off for over 15 years, staying away from white flour, sugar and other processed foods."
– Dee McCaffrey, Chemist & Diet Counselor, Tempe, AZ

Lou & Patricia in Chicago Health Freedom Expo.

PATRICIA CONTINUING BRAGG HEALTH CRUSADE!

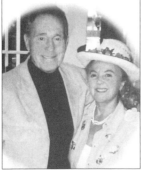

Jack LaLanne with Patricia.

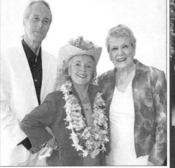

Jon & Elaine LaLanne with Patricia.

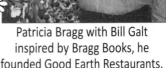

Mother Nature Loves US!

Patricia Bragg with Bill Galt inspired by Bragg Books, he founded Good Earth Restaurants.

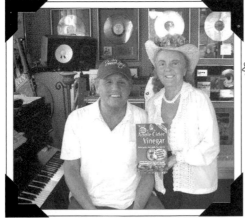

Patricia in studio with famous Beach Boy Bruce Johnston, Bragg follower over 40 years. He played for her their latest records.

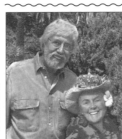

Patricia with Jean-Michel Cousteau Ocean Explorer & Environmentalist. OceanFutures.org

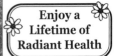

Enjoy a Lifetime of Radiant Health

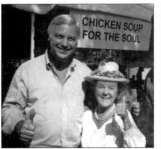

Patricia with Jack Canfield, Bragg follower, Motivational Speaker and Co-Producer of *Chicken Soup For The Soul*.

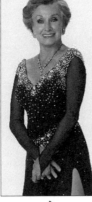

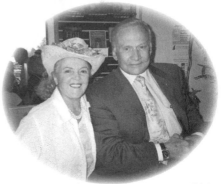

Patricia with Astronaut Buzz Aldrin, celebrating over 50 years since pilot of Apollo 11 first landed on the moon.

Famous Hollywood Actress Cloris Leachman, ardent health follower who sparkled with health and vitality said, *"The Miracle of Fasting Book is a miracle . . . it cured my asthma, my years of arthritis and many other health problems. I praise Paul and Patricia daily for their Health Crusading!"*

PHOTO GALLERY

PAUL & PATRICIA BRAGG HEALTH CRUSADING

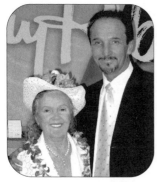

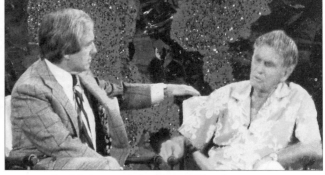

Patricia with Jay Robb.

Paul C. Bragg on the Merv Griffin Show, 1976.

Paul Bragg inspired me many years ago with The Miracle of Fasting Book and his pioneering philosophy on health. His daughter Patricia is a testament to the ageless value of living The Bragg Healthy Lifestyle. – Jay Robb, author of The Fruit Flush

During the many years Patricia worked with her father, she was right beside him, assisting him on Bragg Health Crusades worldwide. They were a great team, when you looked at them, you would see only two people headed in the same healthy direction!

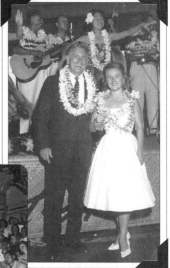

I am a big fan of Paul Bragg. I fast and follow The Bragg Healthy Lifestyle daily. The world and I are blessed with the health teachings of Paul and Patricia Bragg!
– Tony Robbins • TonyRobbins.com

❀ **Dream big, think big and enjoy the many miracles.** ❀

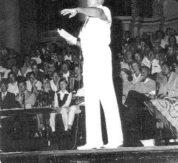

Paul & Daughter Patricia, Royal Hawaiian, Honolulu.

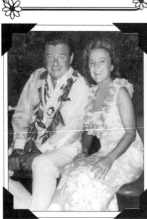

Paul – London Bragg Health Crusade.

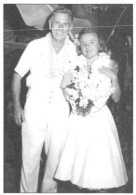

N

Actor Arthur Godfrey with Patricia, in Honolulu celebrating his 79th birthday.

Health Crusaders Paul C. Bragg and daughter Patricia traveled the world spreading health, inspiring millions to renew and revitalize their health.
Bragg Mottos:
3 John 2 and Genesis 6:3

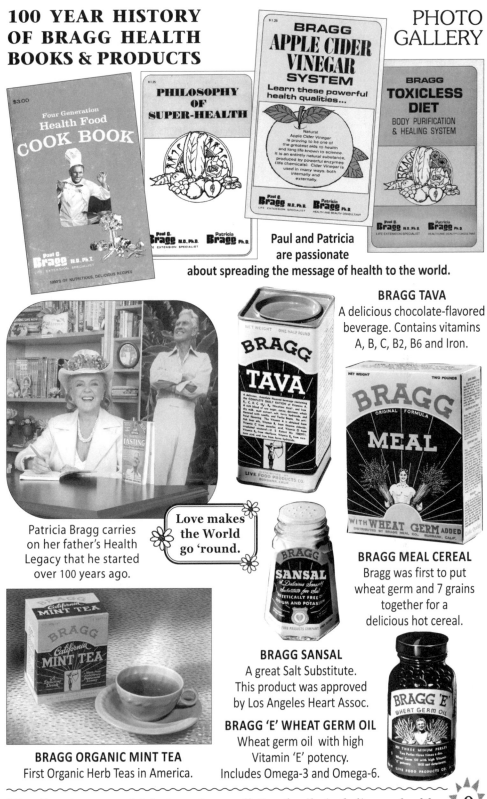

Four Generation Health Food COOK BOOK
$3.00
Paul C. Bragg N.D. Ph.T.
LIFE EXTENSION SPECIALIST
1000'S OF NUTRITIOUS, DELICIOUS RECIPES

PHILOSOPHY OF SUPER-HEALTH
Paul C. Bragg N.D. Ph.D.
LIFE EXTENSION SPECIALIST
Patricia Bragg Ph.D.

BRAGG APPLE CIDER VINEGAR SYSTEM
$1.25
Learn these powerful health qualities...

Natural Apple Cider Vinegar is proving to be one of the greatest aids to health and long life known to science. It is an entirely natural substance, produced by powerful enzymes (life chemicals). Cider Vinegar is used in many ways, both internally and externally.

Paul C. Bragg N.D. Ph.D.
LIFE EXTENSION SPECIALIST
Patricia Bragg Ph.D.
HEALTH AND BEAUTY CONSULTANT

BRAGG TOXICLESS DIET
BODY PURIFICATION & HEALING SYSTEM
Paul C. Bragg N.D. Ph.D.
LIFE EXTENSION SPECIALIST
Patricia Bragg Ph.D.
HEALTH AND BEAUTY CONSULTANT

Paul and Patricia are passionate about spreading the message of health to the world.

Patricia Bragg carries on her father's Health Legacy that he started over 100 years ago.

Love makes the World go 'round.

BRAGG TAVA
A delicious chocolate-flavored beverage. Contains vitamins A, B, C, B2, B6 and Iron.

BRAGG MEAL CEREAL
Bragg was first to put wheat germ and 7 grains together for a delicious hot cereal.

BRAGG SANSAL
A great Salt Substitute. This product was approved by Los Angeles Heart Assoc.

BRAGG 'E' WHEAT GERM OIL
Wheat germ oil with high Vitamin 'E' potency. Includes Omega-3 and Omega-6.

BRAGG ORGANIC MINT TEA
First Organic Herb Teas in America.

"Our lives have completely turned around! Our family is feeling so healthy, we must tell you about it."– Gene & Joan Zollner, parents of 11, Washington

PHOTO GALLERY **Celebrating Years of Health Crusading**

HALL of LEGENDS
Patricia Bragg

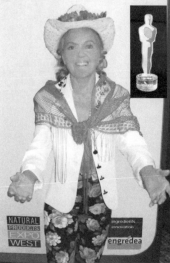

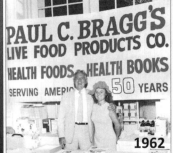

1962

Paul C. Bragg with Patricia, celebrating over 50 years of Bragg Health Products, Books & Crusading worldwide, spreading Health around the world.

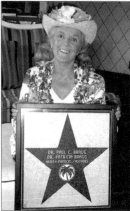

"Palm Spring Walk of Stars" – Patricia with Bragg Star.

Natural Foods Expo in Anaheim with 65,000 attendees from around the world honored Patricia Bragg and her father Paul C. Bragg as treasured Health Food Industry Legends.

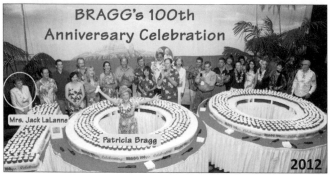

BRAGG's 100th Anniversary Celebration

Mrs. Jack LaLanne

Patricia Bragg

2012

100 Year Anniversary Party celebrated at the Natural Foods Expo in Anaheim

Patricia, Staff & 1,000 Friends celebrated our 100 years of Bragg Healthy Products, Books & Health Crusading! We are proud Pioneers in this Big Health Industry that is helping to keep the world healthier! With Blessings of Health, Peace & Love to You!

Patricia

Bragg Hawaii Exercise Class was founded by Worldwide Health Crusader and Fitness Legend, Dr. Paul C. Bragg. He wanted to create a dynamic, Free Community Exercise Class, and he often taught these classes himself for many years. Patricia Bragg continues her father's health legacy by supporting the Bragg Exercise Class and participates in the class whenever she is in Hawaii.

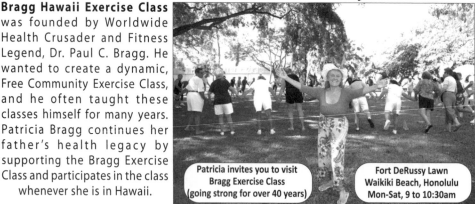

Patricia invites you to visit Bragg Exercise Class (going strong for over 40 years)

Fort DeRussy Lawn Waikiki Beach, Honolulu Mon-Sat, 9 to 10:30am

---

"Please make a record of your family history & background. Take pictures – make **P** *your own 'Photo Gallery'. Take videos – make movies of your children, spouse, mother and father, family gatherings, etc. These memories are precious & important to save for future generations."* – Patricia Bragg

Patricia Bragg Books

BRAGG
HEALTHY
LIFESTYLE

Vital Living at Any Age!

The Lifestyle that Keeps you Ageless
Followed by Millions

PAUL C. BRAGG, N.D., Ph.D.
LIFE EXTENSION SPECIALIST
and
PATRICIA BRAGG
HEALTH CRUSADER & LIFESTYLE EDUCATOR

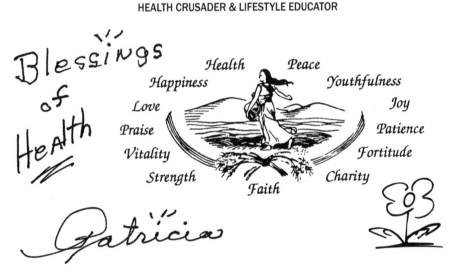

Blessings of Health

Health   Peace
Happiness   Youthfulness
Love   Joy
Praise   Patience
Vitality   Fortitude
Strength   Charity
Faith

Patricia

BECOME
A Health Crusader – for a 100% Healthy World for All!

www.PatriciaBraggBooks.com

BRAGG
HEALTHY
LIFESTYLE

Vital Living at Any Age!

The Lifestyle that Keeps you Ageless
Followed by Millions

PAUL C. BRAGG, N.D., Ph.D.
LIFE EXTENSION SPECIALIST
and
PATRICIA BRAGG
HEALTH CRUSADER & LIFESTYLE EDUCATOR

Visit our website:
www.PatriciaBraggBooks.com

Thirty-Eighth Edition MMXXI
ISBN: 978-0-87790-082-5

Library of Congress Cataloging-in-Publication Data on file with publisher

Published in the United States
HEALTH SCIENCE
7127 Hollister Avenue, Suite 25A, Box 249, Santa Barbara, CA 93117
Toll-Free: (833) 408-1122

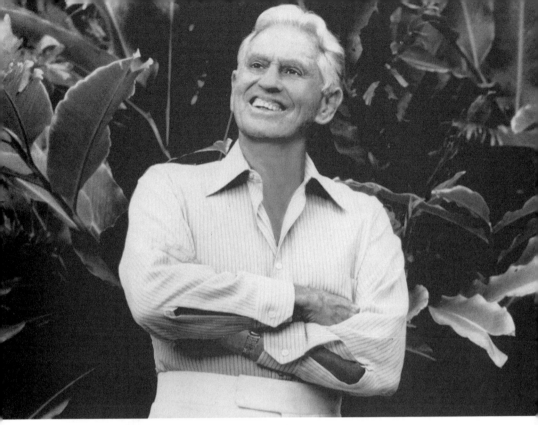

PAUL C. BRAGG, N.D., Ph.D.
World's Leading Healthy Lifestyle Authority

Paul C. Bragg's daughter Patricia and their wonderful, healthy members of the Bragg *Longer Life, Health and Happiness Club* exercised daily on the beautiful Fort DeRussy lawn, at famous Waikiki Beach in Honolulu, Hawaii. On Saturday there were often health lectures on how to live a long, healthy life! The group averaged 50 to 75 per day, depending on the season. From December to March it can go up to 125. Its dedicated leaders carried on the class for over 43 years. Thousands visited the club from around the world and carried the Bragg Health and Fitness Crusade to friends and relatives back home.

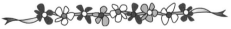

Your body is a non-stop living system, in constant motion 24 hours daily, cleaning, repairing, healing and growing. – Patricia Bragg

To maintain good health, normal weight and increase the good life of radiant health, joy and happiness, the body must be exercised properly (stretching, walking, jogging, biking, swimming, deep breathing, good posture) and nourished with healthy foods. – Paul C. Bragg, N.D., Ph.D.

iii

❀ Cautionary Note and Disclaimer ❀

The information provided here is for educational purposes only. Any decision on your part to read, listen and use this information is your personal choice. The information in this book is not meant to be used to diagnose, prescribe or treat any illness. Please discuss any changes you wish to make to your medical treatment with a qualified, licensed health care provider.

If you are taking medication to control your blood sugar or blood pressure, you may need to reduce the dosage if you significantly restrict your carbohydrate intake. This is best done under the care and supervision of an experienced and qualified licensed health care provider. Anyone who has any other serious illness such as cardiovascular disease, cancer, kidney or liver disease needs to exercise caution if making dietary changes. You should consult your physician for guidance. If you are pregnant or lactating, you should not overly restrict protein or fat intake. Also, young children and teens have much more demanding nutrient needs and should NOT have their protein or fat intake overly restricted.

The information presented in this book is in no way intended as medical advice or a substitute for medical counseling. It is intended only to provide the opinions and ideas of the authors. It is sold with the understanding that the authors are not engaged in rendering medical, health or any other kind of professional services in this book. The reader should consult his or her medical doctor, or any other competent professional, before adopting any of the suggestions in this book, or drawing inferences from it.

The authors disclaim any responsibility for any liability, loss or risk, personal or otherwise, which is incurred as a consequence, directly or indirectly, of the use and application of the contents of this book.

Please consult your physician before beginning this program, and use all of the information the authors suggest in conjunction with the guidance and care of your physician. Your physician should be aware of all medical conditions that you may have, as well as medications and supplements you are taking.

BRAGG
HEALTHY
LIFESTYLE
Vital Living at Any Age!

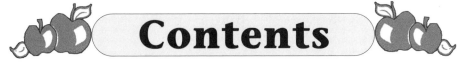

To preserve health is a moral and religious duty, for health is the basis for all social virtues. We can no longer be as useful when not well.
– Dr. Samuel Johnson, Father of Dictionaries, 1709-1784

Contents

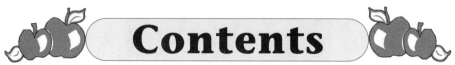

Contents

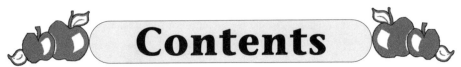

Contents

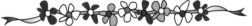

Love is the sun shining in us to sparkle our lives! – Patricia Bragg

*Bragg Health Books are silent health teachers and your friends –
never tiring, ready night or day to help guide you to super health!*

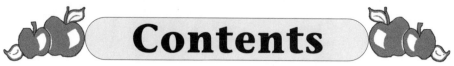

Contents

*The more natural food you eat, the more you'll enjoy radiant health and
be able to promote the higher life of love and brotherhood. – Patricia Bragg*

*A fool thinks he needs no advice, but a wise man listens & learns from others.
– Proverbs 12:15*

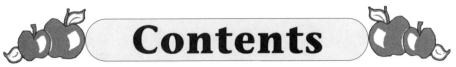

Contents

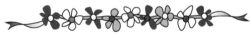

When you sell a man a book you don't just sell him paper and ink, you sell him a whole new life! There's heaven and earth in a real book. The real purpose of books is to inspire the mind into doing its own thinking. – Christopher Morley

Kindness should be a frame of mind in which we are alert to every chance: to do, to give, to share and to be kind and loving. – Patricia Bragg

We shall never know all the good that a simple smile can do.
– Mother Teresa

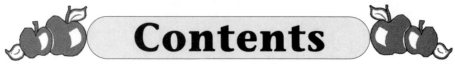

Contents

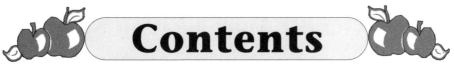

Contents

*It's important for each of us to have a special private area for ourselves –
a place set aside for daydreaming, reading, meditation and prayer to help
us rejuvenate from everyday life! This area can include anything that is
meaningful and inspiring, including music you like. It should be a special
place in your home, garden, etc. where you go to relax and reconnect with
your inner self – your secret garden where you can grow and be nurtured.*
– UC Berkeley Wellness Newsletter • www.BerkeleyWellness.com

Introduction to Your Exciting New Life!

Life is the Miracle of Miracles

You hold the miracle of miracles right now in the palm of your hand. You have the treasure of precious life! Think what that means to you. You are a living, breathing person! Life is the most priceless treasure on this earth. You have that treasure. Within you lies the mental power to be anything you want to be! You have a reasoning, logical mind. Within your being you have the kingdom of heaven. Find that heaven and you have reached bliss-consciousness. You'll have found heaven on earth and life becomes so precious and wonderful!

If you want more health, energy and a longer life, you will have to plan, plot and start creating, becoming and shaping your life! Look ahead. Have firm plans for living your life. Actually envision your future. You may change those plans and visions, but have them you must! Your creative force deep within you must reach out toward a brighter future if you want to become one with the healthy flow for an exciting, fulfilling life! Your entire mind and being will be super energized in the process to go for your future goals and dreams.

Make Your Body Worry–Proof

As usual, the Greeks created this perfect phrase for this human interrelationship: *A strong mind in a strong body.* No one has said it better. If you're mentally upset, you can walk miles – but if you're physically sick, clear, constructive thinking is virtually impossible. By raising your physical health standards, your mental abilities will increase accordingly. Be on healthy terms with your body, mind and soul to fully balance and enjoy your life, physically, mentally, emotionally and spiritually.

(Copy page, cut out Patricia's Angel Strip, for you to fold and keep in wallet.)

Angel to Protect & Guide You

*Here's your own "Pocket Angel" to be with you 24/7
night and day to guide, protect, and show you
right from wrong, and help you heal your life
– physically, mentally, emotionally and spiritually
with Angel Love.*

Chapter 1

Bragg Healthy Lifestyle Vital Living at Any Age!

The Bragg Toxicless Diet, Body Purification and Healing System

This *course of life instruction* is for those who want to learn how to improve, maintain and extend their health and live to a healthy 120 years! Millions worldwide have benefited and achieved super health from the message spread by my father and myself. Now it's your turn to get started with The Bragg Healthy Lifestyle!

We are Health Crusading Pioneers and our passion is sharing health with you, our readers and health friends! **Soon after you start, the benefits from our health teachings will become amazingly apparent in your life** and you will begin enjoying all of their wonder-working miracles!

This mind-opening, life-changing book will help you find and draw upon your body's own natural resources of health, energy and youthfulness! It teaches you to free yourself from the health wreckers that are destroying your health! It shows you how to flush out the toxins that cause most health problems. It also helps you eliminate stress, strain, tension and fatigue. Best of all, **it helps you develop sparkling new supplies of health, zest and energy for a long, happy and fulfilled life!**

There is no reason why after reading this book, with your new understanding of how to live The Bragg Healthy Lifestyle, that you can't live a longer, happier, healthier life!

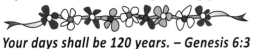

Your days shall be 120 years. – Genesis 6:3

You are what you eat, drink, breathe, think, say and do. – Patricia Bragg

---

So this morning begin by eating God's natural foods, drink pure water, think positive thoughts, affirm aloud, take healthy action and tomorrow will be brighter, happier and healthier than you ever dreamed possible!
– Robert Anthony Schuller, former pastor, Crystal Cathedral

The Toxicless Diet, Body Purification And Healing System Fully Explained

First, we want it definitely understood that this system does not claim to cure disease. No system can "cure" disease. Only the internal functions of your own body can banish disease! The human body is self-cleansing, self-repairing and self-healing! You break a bone, the doctor sets the bone and puts it into a cast. The broken bone knits together again. After a certain number of weeks, the bone is again as strong as it was before the break – sometimes even stronger! There is no special diet, no special foods, no pill, no injection or prescription that can "cure" or mend a broken bone. The internal healing forces are within every human body – these are what rebuild and heal the broken bone!

Only Mother Nature Cures!

Burn this into your consciousness: Only Mother Nature Cures! Every human body has a special built-in healing mechanism. You cut your hand and three to five stitches might be required to close the wound. The doctor cleans, then stitches and bandages the wound and can do no more. Now the miraculous healing mechanism of your body starts mending the wound.

Discover and Guard Your Body's Vital Force

To simplify this explanation of The Toxicless Diet, Body Purification and Healing System, we are going to call this vital healing power "Vital Force!" All of us must have this Vital Force energy in order to stay alive! When the Vital Force is completely exhausted, there is death. Many people live at a very low rate of "physical vibration" because they have a very low amount of Vital Force. Then there are people who live a healthy lifestyle every day who enjoy a high rate of physical vibration with high energy! Their Vital Force is high!

Man's body was created according to the laws of physics and chemistry, which are the Creator's laws. They never vary. His law is written upon every nerve, muscle and faculty which has been entrusted to us.
– Henry W. Vollmer, M.D.

Every day of your life you meet people with a high amount of Vital Force. On the other hand, every day you also see tired, exhausted, nervous, frustrated people full of aches, pains, diseases, stresses and tensions. Most of these people are prematurely old . . . they appear and act older than their calendar years! People with a low quota of Vital Force have a low resistance to infectious diseases – they are the people who have frequent colds, flu, strep throat and many other disorders! They are the people who are chronically tired, suffering from what is often called "Chronic Fatigue Syndrome" and Epstein-Barr. They are the people with poor memories who are full of aches and pains. They are lifeless, pale and often anemic.

Lack of Vital Force Brings on Enervation!

With the Vital Force energy at a low ebb enervation takes over. When enervation takes over physical troubles start to multiply! Remember first and foremost, we are miraculous instruments. In order for our bodies to be "in tune" and operate 100% efficiently, there must be adequate Vital Force and a Healthy Lifestyle! It's needed to keep the eliminative organs removing the accumulating toxins and wastes from our bodies daily! A clean internal body operates happily and more efficiently.

3

There you have it – the secret of life in a nutshell! The body accumulates a certain amount of toxic waste from food you eat and drink. As food passes through the gastrointestinal tract, the great body intelligence selects nutrients it needs and the waste is passed out of the body. This squeeze and push function requires large amounts of Vital Force. If a person has low Vital Force, food wastes don't pass out of the body in normal time, then toxins build up causing problems!

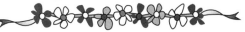

Love makes the world go 'round, and it's everlasting when it's written with caring, loving advice that will improve and enrich your life! This is why my father and I love sharing with you the health wisdoms which can be with you on your long life's journey. Our books on health, fitness and longevity go 'round the world spreading health, peace of mind and love! – Patricia Bragg

 Behind every wise, successful person is themselves.
– American Proverb

The body has a warm temperature of 98.6°F. If food wastes remain too long in the gastrointestinal tract, daily toxic poisons build up. Then auto-intoxication and putrefaction starts to set in. Toxic poisons are then thrown back into the bloodstream and you start to self-poison and self-pollute! The many dangerous effects of this toxic poison being thrown back into the bloodstream can become devastating and deadly!

Enervation and Disease: Cause and Effect

Mother Nature always gives warnings when toxic poisons start to build up in the bloodstream – such as headaches. Some ache, others throb and then there are the worst of all, severe migraine headaches! There are also many other symptoms of auto-intoxication – nausea, mental depression, irritability, stress and tension. The full list of symptoms is too long to enumerate here. Toxic Enervation slows down the eliminative functions not only of bowels, but kidneys, skin and lungs. Our bodies cannot efficiently eliminate accumulating toxic wastes when our "Vital Force" is in a sluggish, low vibration, enervated condition!

For every effect there must be a cause! All disease conditions are effects of enervation! The basic cause of enervation is poor diet and unhealthy lifestyle. The average food of civilization has been so perverted and robbed of life and energy that most of its vital nutrients have been removed! You cannot expect to build a high healthy Vital Force on poor fuel. Most humans suffer from chronic malnutrition. The prefix "mal" means ill or bad. So malnutrition means ill nutrition and in plain words adds up to bad health!

The preservation of health is a duty. Few seem conscious that there is such a thing as physical morality. – Herbert Spencer

A healthy body is a guest-chamber for the soul; a sick body is a prison.
– Francis Bacon, 1st Viscount, Philosopher, Scientist, Author, 16th Century

I cannot overstate the importance of the habit of quiet prayer and meditation for more health of body, mind and spirit.
"In quietness shall be your strength." – Isaiah 30:15

Bad Nutrition –
#1 Cause of Sickness
"Diet-related diseases account for 68% of all deaths."
– Dr. C. Everett Koop

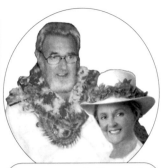

Dr. Koop & Patricia
World Health Conference in Hawaii

America's former Surgeon General and our friend, said this in his famous 1988 landmark report on nutrition and health in America. People don't die of infectious conditions as such, but of malnutrition that allows the germs to get a foothold in sickly bodies. Also, bad nutrition is usually the cause of non-infectious, fatal or degenerative conditions. When the body has its full nutrition quota of vitamin and minerals, including potassium, it's almost impossible for germs to get a foothold in a healthy, powerful bloodstream and tissues!

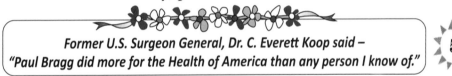

Former U.S. Surgeon General, Dr. C. Everett Koop said –
"Paul Bragg did more for the Health of America than any person I know of."

5

Foods Can Make or Break Your Health!

People are so steeped in their health-breaking habits of eating that they think some mysterious potion will do away with all of their physical miseries! They want to circumvent all their bad eating habits. They don't even realize that the food they eat can either make you a physical wreck or can give you Health Supreme!

There Are No Miracle Cures Except Those Performed by Mother Nature!

This brings us to the Great Law of Compensation. You cannot get something for nothing! The precious health we teach and write about is a Super-High Health that you must earn by living a healthy lifestyle! No one can cure you . . . NO ONE CAN BANISH YOUR AILMENTS! Health works with this great Law of Compensation. **Health building requires individual discipline!** Your miracle mind and *brain* (computer) must take over the operation of your precious body, because flesh is dumb!

You can put anything into your mouth and swallow it. Only a clear, intelligent, reasoning mind will wisely supervise what is put in the stomach! Always remember that what you eat and drink today will be walking and talking tomorrow. Food is your fuel! Healthy food makes fuel that gives good performance!

"Thy Food Will Be Thy Remedy!" – Hippocrates

In 400 B.C., on the Chios Island (now Khios) in classical Greece, Hippocrates, the bearded physician-teacher-Father of Medicine, sat in the shade of beautiful trees on the hillside. There Hippocrates taught and enlightened his medical students with these brilliant, factual and ageless words of wisdom so needed today!

Your Food Will Be Your Remedy . . . No one, to date, has more eloquently described a healthy way of life! This entire Toxicless Diet, Body Purification and Healing System is based on this one vital truth! This System is based on the principle that with healthy foods and fasting you can cleanse, purify and rebuild your body and find perfect health again. Yes, food can be your medicine!

My father, over the course of his entire, long lifetime, proved that within fruits and vegetables are the amazing natural remedies for most of man's physical problems.

Wisely, Hippocrates, the Father of Medicine, treated his patients with amazing raw Apple Cider Vinegar because he recognized its powerful cleansing and healing qualities. It's a naturally occurring antibiotic and antiseptic that fights germs, viruses, bacteria and even mold.

The medical profession insists that it strives to emulate the Father of all Physicians. Indeed, it requires its Practitioners to take the Hippocratic Oath, one of the most sublime declarations of lofty ethics ever written. Yet today there are thousands of dedicated bacteriologists,

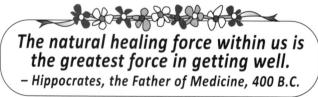

The natural healing force within us is the greatest force in getting well.
– Hippocrates, the Father of Medicine, 400 B.C.

Everything in excess is opposed by nature. – Hippocrates

pharmaceutical researchers and chemists sitting in gleaming laboratories throughout the world, busily turning out synthetic, so-called "magic" drug panaceas for every human misery. Unlike the wise Hippocrates, their unwise battle cry appears to be: "Thy remedy shall be our newly invented wonder drug."

You Become What You Eat and Drink

Because the human body is the most powerful miracle instrument, it can take years and years of the cruelest punishment from an unhealthy lifestyle. Then comes the day of reckoning when the body reaches its capacity for being loaded down with unhealthy fats, grease, sugar, salt, preserved, refined and junk fast foods that produce sick, clogged bloodstreams! Then disease strikes with all its powerful force! Cataracts blind and blur the vision. Arthritis cripples and stiffens joints. Ears go deaf. Varicose veins cripple the legs. Ulcers form in the stomach and intestines. Piles and deadly fissures attack the rectum. These are just a few of over 4,000 crippling diseases that can make life a living hell while on this Earth!

These tragic things do not just happen . . . it's again the Eternal Law of Compensation at work. Mother Nature is a hard taskmaster, disobey her laws and soon she will give you punishment that is beyond human comprehension.

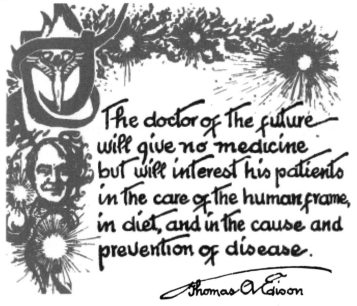

The doctor of the future will give no medicine but will interest his patients in the care of the human frame, in diet, and in the cause and prevention of disease.

Thomas A. Edison

"Fast Relief" Claims Misguide Americans

Look at the TV commercials – the old and new remedies flash on the screen. We have all heard many claims of – get fast relief for headaches, with this remedy or the other. Fast relief for acid stomach, heartburn and indigestion. If your joints and muscles hurt, take this fast remedy. Not only TV, but also radio, newspapers, magazines and the web are full of remedies for all kinds of human physical and mental ailments.

The unhealthy and anxiety-ridden Americans by the millions obey the persuasive messages of TV ads that cost the drug companies millions. People are led to believe they can purchase health and energy at stores in bottles filled with miracle drugs, powders, liquids and pills. They don't know that true health can be found only by obeying Mother Nature's Healthy Lifestyle Laws.

Ailing, sickly people today are constantly looking for an instant "cure-all", miracle substance that will restore their lost health, energy and youth! **This Toxicless Diet, Body Purification and Healing System is the intelligent way to follow the clear-cut Laws of Mother Nature.**

8

Don't Clog the Pipes of Your Body

Your body is really a miracle plumbing system. You are made up of small pipes, medium-sized pipes and large pipes like the gastrointestinal tract, which is 30 feet long. Through the gastrointestinal pipe, from the mouth to the rectum, flows all the food and drink you consume.

There is a great miracle muscular system within the gastrointestinal tract that propels the food slowly down and outward. To keep this muscular action efficient, the food we eat must contain bulk, moisture and lubrication. This is supplied by coarse raw vegetables such as cabbage (red and green), beets, broccoli, carrots, celery, turnips and radishes, etc. All raw vegetables contribute to strengthen the muscular action along the gastrointestinal tract. We call raw vegetables and raw fruits "Nature's Broom." They are absolutely necessary if you want to

The human body has one ability not possessed by any machine –
the body has the ability to repair and heal itself. – George W. Crile

enjoy higher health and longevity! Even the American Cancer Society and the United States Surgeon General agree: eating fruits and vegetables is important for the prevention of cancer.

In our opinion, every disease – no matter what its scientific name – is basically caused by the clogging of the human pipe system! Any localized symptom is therefore merely the result of a local clogging by the buildup of toxic waste poisons at that particular point. Any part of the pipe system can become clogged. The #1 killer of them all in America is "Heart Disease," the accumulation of matter (toxins, cholesterol, fats) that clogs the cardiovascular system and the heart! Yes, this is the world's most deadly disease – hardening of the arteries. The vicious toxic material that hardens the arteries can completely block them so that your vital life-giving oxygenated blood cannot pass through. Hardening of the arteries does not happen overnight; it takes a long time to develop this fatal condition! Yet, recent studies show that some people start to get hardening of the arteries at a very early age. The cause is their unhealthy lifestyle!

Learn to Apply Health Lessons from History

Premature hardening of the arteries was observed even as early as the Korean War, when 350 U.S. soldiers were closely examined after death. These were young men, between ages of 18 and 28. Autopsies revealed that all of them had a certain amount of hardening in their arteries! There is little doubt that these young men had, since childhood, been fed on the Standard (unhealthy) American Diet (S.A.D.). They ate meals high in fats, meats, sugared cereals, desserts and other highly processed foods. Their devitalized, highly refined diet was heavily loaded with salt, saturated fats and refined white sugar. (Widely used today is a toxic sugar substitute called aspartame. See page 64 and web: *www.drkevinsdailydose.com*). Many doctors and studies agree refined white sugar, salt and saturated fats lead to diabetes, heart conditions, hardening of the arteries and premature ageing.

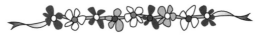

We live not upon what we eat, but upon what we digest. – Abernethy

All of their lives these young men had been fed on commercially hardened fats of all kinds. They had eaten smoked and brine-cured meats such as bacon, ham, sausage, luncheon meats and all other kinds of preserved meats. They were also heavy users of processed fast foods containing table salt (*a harmful inorganic sodium*) and toxic preservatives. The naturally occurring organic sodium found in foods and seaweeds are the best source! (*Celtic salt in small amounts is acceptable if desired.*)

Why Does Premature Ageing Happen?

In other words, these young soldiers grew up on a diet of hardened fats, cholesterol and toxin-producing foods. As a result of their unhealthy diet they started to develop cardiovascular degenerative disease before the age of 30! Remember, clogging of the human pipe system can start when a youngster! This is the reason why many people prematurely age! It's sad that people age way before their time. In our world travels we find many people who look and act 20 to 30 years older than their chronological age! Why? It's their unhealthy lifestyles!

10

Forget Calendar Years – Be Ageless!

Just because a person lives to be 60, 70, 80, 90 or more is no reason to believe that they should suffer from any degenerative disease such as hardening of the arteries. Most people's thinking is controlled by mob psychology. The average person has been trained to think falsely that as the years go by you are supposed to get old, decline and sadly, deteriorate in body and mind. *"Age brings on troubles,"* they have been told and that is exactly what they believe!

You cannot control your chronological years, but with The Bragg Healthy Lifestyle, you can most assuredly control your biological age . . . in fact you can almost hold it to a standstill! A healthy life is wonderful and fulfilling! It's exciting to be active, healthy, alert and to be of help and of service to this world! My father and I love sharing with you – our readers – this great message of The Bragg Healthy Lifestyle in this book! **Please open your mind, heart and soul and realize that you can be in control of your health and enjoy a healthy, long life!**

Health Road or Sickness Road?
Which Road Will You Take?

Health, like freedom and peace, lasts as long as we exert ourselves to maintain it. You must make your choice! It's almost exclusively in your hands whether you enjoy a healthy, vigorous life to a ripe old age or live out a half-alive, non-energetic existence with premature breakdown of health. You can decide to travel the average (unhealthy) road. But seldom will someone tell you the errors of this way. No one will stop you! You will have lots of company.

Again let us give you a serious health warning . . . remember that you are going to pay dearly for every sin you commit against your body! The wages of sin are physical suffering, aches, pains and often a premature early death! Start living The Bragg Healthy Lifestyle today, to ensure a bright, healthy, fulfilled future!

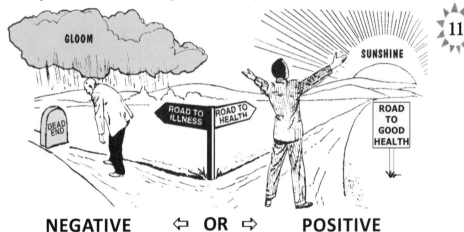

NEGATIVE ⇦ OR ⇨ POSITIVE

The choice of which road to take is up to you.

You alone decide whether to reach a dead end or live a healthy lifestyle for a long, healthy, happy, active life. – Paul C. Bragg, N.D., Ph.D.

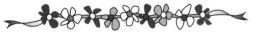

The first wealth is your health. – Ralph Waldo Emerson

It is sad that many people go through life committing partial slow suicide destroying their health, youth, beauty, talents, energies and creative qualities. Indeed, to learn how to be good to oneself is often more difficult than to learn how to be good to others.
– Paul C. Bragg, N.D., Ph.D.

Mother Nature Loves You To Enjoy Her Beauty

Let me look upward
into the branches
Of the towering oak
And know that it grew
slowly and well.

Give me, amidst
the confusion
of my day
The calmness of the
everlasting hills.

Let me pause
to look at a flower,
to smell a rose —
God's autograph,
to chat with a friend,
to read a few lines
from a good book.

Break the tensions
of my nerves
With the soothing music
of singing streams
and gentle rains
That live in
my memory.

Follow steps of the godly,
and stay on the right path
to enjoy life to the fullest.
— Proverbs 2:20-21

12

Open your eyes to behold wondrous things out of Thy law.
— Psalm 119:18

Chapter 2

Proven Steps of Wisdom to Agelessness And Longevity

Enjoy Long Life – We Are Always Renewed

We believe it is possible to live in a perfect state of agelessness. Let's reason it out together. Every 3 months you get an entirely new bloodstream, so it is not the bloodstream that gets old. Every 11 months, every cell in the body has renewed itself . . . so you have a practically new body every 11 months. Every 2 years you get an entirely new bone structure, so in 3 years you are really born again . . . the renewal process has taken place! Now, if you keep the body clean and purified by eating a diet that continually cleanses the body, how can you get sick? How can you get old?

We have met in our many years of travel hundreds of people 100 and more years old; their eyes were perfect, they had no hardening of the arteries, no blindness, no aches and pains. Most of these people lived their early lives in rural settings where they never ate refined and processed foods. They lived active lives on simple, natural, healthy foods from their own surroundings.

13

If these people had known about The Bragg Healthy Lifestyle they could have controlled their life and the ageing process indefinitely and lived even longer!

Why Die Before Your Time?

Read in the Bible where some people lived 900 and more years in a state of ageless grace! Of course the skeptics will scoff at these ages and say, "They recorded time differently than we do." But they have not studied these ancient people's habits. They lived on foods that

Don't procrastinate and keep waiting for "the right moment."
Today – take action, plan, plot and follow through with your goals,
dreams and healthy living! You will be a winner in life when you Captain
your life to success! – Patricia Bragg, Pioneer Health Crusader

did not obstruct and clog the pipe system. This was the only thing that kept them alive – a clean body, free from clogging, encumbrances and obstructions. And that is exactly what this *Course of Instruction* is going to give you – a clean, healthy body! The Bragg Healthy Lifestyle will help you keep the toxic poisons flushing out of the body. Who knows? You, our reader and new health friend, may live 100 years or more in abundant health by living this healthy, active and vital lifestyle! We want this for all of you – a long, happy, healthy and fulfilling life!

Remember that death is brought to the body when it's so saturated and bogged down with stored toxic poison that it can no longer function to maintain life! Start now to be a good health captain of your entire life! Don't allow toxins into your body. Keep it clean and pure so you will reap super health, energy and enjoy longevity!

The Garden of Eden

14 We believe man once lived in a tropical paradise. In all our research and study we have come to the definite conclusion that man once lived in a *"Garden of Eden,"* and his diet consisted of raw fruits and raw vegetables and some lightly cooked vegetables. We believe that the man of Eden ate many green leafy vegetables, and that he ate nuts and seeds.

Now we want to clarify this whole statement so we will not be misunderstood. We believe that man lived in this tropical paradise and that at no time did they have to worry about being cold. They could lie down at night and sleep without any discomfort or chill. This is the true state of man. But then we find this was to change because of the approach of the Ice Ages. All over the world lifestyles were altered many times by these climate changes. As man was forced to live in colder areas, the variety of fruits and vegetables available to him was naturally reduced and limited to seasonal crops.

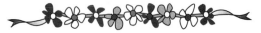

Be your own Health Captain and do what needs to be done for your health!

Follow Mother Nature and God – rewards are great! – Patricia Bragg

Unhealthy Lifestyle, Milk & Meat Shorten Life!

Now allow us to repeat this to make it clear in your mind. When man lived in his tropical paradise on a diet of natural, organically grown fruits and vegetables, he was constantly detoxifying and purifying his body. He lived every day on *The Toxicless Diet, Body Purification and Healing System*. Most lived a long life, free from aches and pains, diseases, premature ageing and senility.

When man left his paradise, it necessitated his venturing into different climates. Then his diet was changed by necessity towards the eating of more grain foods like wheat, barley, oats, rye, maize and millet. He also learned to cultivate rice, lentils and beans of all varieties, which he dried and stored for long periods of time. Having his fruit and vegetable selection greatly reduced, he turned to the killing of animals for meat and the collecting of birds' eggs. In time he found he could domesticate animals like the cow, goat and fowl. Not only did these provide him with ready meat, but he also had a fresh egg supply, and it wasn't long before he mastered the milking of the cow, goat and the sheep.

From this milk he learned to make butter, cheese and other dairy products. So, from a predominantly healthy alkaline diet, climate changes forced man to slowly change his eating habits until his diet was one heavy in starch, proteins, fats and acids. Meat is heavy in uric acid, which is quite toxic! Meat also carries visible and invisible fats (clogging waxy substance called cholesterol), along with any toxic waste, viruses, germs, chemicals, drugs, hormones, antibiotics (now given to animals) and diseases in circulation in animal's body at time of slaughter and demise. See website: *www.GoVeg.com.*

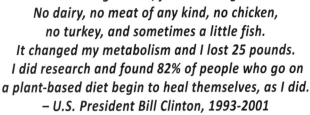

I live on vegetables, fruits and legumes.
No dairy, no meat of any kind, no chicken,
no turkey, and sometimes a little fish.
It changed my metabolism and I lost 25 pounds.
I did research and found 82% of people who go on
a plant-based diet begin to heal themselves, as I did.
– U.S. President Bill Clinton, 1993-2001

The World is Our Human Classroom

People in the world's industrialized countries eat lots of fresh meat and also all kinds of smoked, salted and preserved meats. Today people worldwide eat many products made with refined white sugar and now the toxic sugar substitute – aspartame (page 64; *diet colas and soft drinks, candy, desserts, pastries*), refined white flour (*breads, doughnuts, pizza*), white rice and processed cheeses, etc. There are over 2,800 toxic chemical additives to color, preserve and stabilize refined, processed foods!

Sadly, We Live in a Toxic World!

In the United States, which is highly representative of these so-called civilized countries, 3.9 billion prescriptions are filled by a white-coated chemist at one of over 250,000 pharmacies in the United States! The staggering cost of these drugs and chemicals that come in many colored tablets, capsules and powders amounts to over a shocking $325 billion a year!

16

When people see their teeth and those of their children with cavities, in utter despair they start to put deadly fluorides in their drinking water, falsely believing that this will keep their teeth perfect and healthy. Read Bragg Book *Water – The Shocking Truth*. We want to share with you the importance of drinking 8 glasses of distilled water daily – nature's great cleanser and purifier that helps operate all your internal machinery!

Please decide now to begin your Bragg Healthy Lifestyle Journey to Higher, Total Health for Total Wellness!
"One step is the beginning of a 10,000 mile journey."

When you live The Bragg Healthy Lifestyle you can activate your own powerful internal defense arsenal and maintain it at top efficiency. However, if you continue with unhealthy diet and lifestyle habits, then it is harder for your body to fight off illness! – Paul C. Bragg, N.D., Ph.D.

Our habits, good or bad, are something we can control.
– Dr. Edward Julius Stieglitz, author, "Geriatric Medicine" 1954

You Can Create Your Own Garden of Eden

My father and I want you to know we have no illusions that there is any place left in the world that could be called 100% perfect. But if you want to be well and live long, **you must work to create your own paradise to the best of your ability wherever you live!** You should strive to live in the most environmentally pure and safe surroundings as possible! Drink only distilled or reverse osmosis-purified water. Eat organic fruits and vegetables. Buy and use air purifiers when needed for home, office and even for your car. This is what we do wherever we live. When possible we have organic vegetable gardens, fruit trees and flowers to create our own Garden of Eden!

This is what The Bragg Healthy Lifestyle is going to do for you. It will inspire and help you establish – wherever you are – your own Garden of Eden! We can't expect to have the exact health, vitality and long life that our brothers and sisters enjoyed in the original Garden of Eden. But we can strive through careful control of our diet, and the purifying and flushing out and eliminating altogether the vicious toxic poisons that are causing us illness, suffering and premature ageing. Naturally there will be some compromises to make. America has had many generations of eating a S.A.D. diet of processed, highly refined and unhealthy foods! **It's important to begin the trip back to your Garden of Eden slowly, wisely and cautiously! You can do it – start now!**

We want you to live a long, healthy, happy, fit life! Decide daily that you want to feel strong, vigorous and that you will banish your aches, pains and tiredness! It's up to you! We pray nightly for all our friends and Bragg readers to be guided down the righteous path of healthy living through these written words – that never tire and can be with you night or day – just for the reading!

Men do not die, they kill themselves. – Seneca, Roman Philosopher 4 B.C.

Uninformed men, when pampered with meat and dairy products are much more irritable, mean and cruel in their tempers than those who live chiefly on fruits and vegetables. – William Smellie, 1780

The First Six Steps To Begin The Bragg Healthy Lifestyle

• Detox • Analyze Your Health
• Transition Diet • Healing Crisis
• Environment • No "Heavy" Breakfast

Step 1: Detox – Rid Yourself of Toxic Foods

The beginning of this program must start with your avoiding the foods and drinks that dangerously clog, obstruct and throw waste into the human pipe system, the body's organs and cells. Study the *Foods to Avoid List* on next page. Some people have stronger constitutions than others. People often make the statement to us that "My Grandfather is 88 and smokes, drinks alcohol and eats any food he wants to, and he is still living!" We have to listen to this occasionally because there are the lucky few who inherit a body that has wide arteries and wide veins. They are born with a capacity to burn poisons three times faster than most! Remember this: when a person who is now 88 years old was born, 86,000 others were also and he is the lone survivor. One out of 86,000 is not a good percentage!

Now, if that man had known about The Toxicless Diet, Body Purification and Healing System and had kept toxic materials down to a minimum, he might have lived to be 150! We have met many healthy men and women over 100 years of age. Start now to discard forever the so-called foods that are highly refined and potentially harmful to your health! See list on next page what uninformed humans put into their bodies.

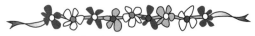

What you eat and drink becomes your body chemistry!
You Must Eat Healthy to Become Healthy!

 Remember, you are punished by your bad habits of living.
– Paul C. Bragg, N.D., Ph.D., Originator Health Stores

Eat not for pleasure thou may find therein; but eat to increase
thy strength and health; eat to preserve the life
thou hast received from Heaven. – Confucius

Avoid These Processed, Refined, Harmful Foods:

Once you realize the harm caused to your body by unhealthy refined, chemicalized, deficient foods, you'll want to eliminate "killer" foods:

- **Refined sugar / artificial sweeteners** (toxic aspartame) or their products such as jams, jellies, preserves, marmalades, yogurts, ice cream, sherbets, Jello, cake, candy, cookies, all chewing gum, colas and diet drinks, pies, pastries, and all sugared fruit juices and fruits canned in sugar syrup. (Health Stores have delicious healthy replacements, such as Stevia, raw honey, 100% maple syrup, and agave nectar, so seek and buy the best).

- **White flour products** such as white bread, wheat-white bread, enriched flours, rye bread that has white flour in it, dumplings, biscuits, buns, gravy, pasta, pancakes, waffles, soda crackers, pizza, ravioli, pies, pastries, cakes, cookies, prepared and commercial puddings and ready-mix bakery products. Most are made with dangerous (oxy-cholesterol) powdered milk and powdered eggs. (Health Stores have a variety of 100% non-GMO whole grain organic products, breads, chips, crackers, pastas, desserts).

- **Salted foods,** such as pretzels, corn chips, potato chips, crackers and nuts.

- **Refined white rice** and pearl barley. • **Fried fast foods.** • **Indian ghee.**

- **Refined dry processed cereals** that are sugared, such as cornflakes, etc.

- **Foods that contain Olestra,** palm and cottonseed oil.

- **Peanuts and peanut butter** that contain hydrogenated, hardened oils and any peanuts with mold and all molds that can cause allergies.

- **Margarine** – combines heart-deadly trans-fatty acids and saturated fats.

- **Saturated fats and hydrogenated oils** – enemies that clog the arteries.

- **Coffee, soft drinks, teas, alcohol, sugared juices** – even if decaffeinated.

- **Fresh pork / products.** • **Fried, fatty, greasy meats.** • **Irradiated** GMO foods.

- **Smoked meats,** such as ham, bacon, sausage and all smoked fish.

- **Luncheon meats,** hot dogs, salami, bologna, corned beef, pastrami and packaged meats containing dangerous sodium nitrate or nitrite.

- **Dried fruits** containing sulphur dioxide – a toxic preservative.

- **Chickens, turkeys and meats injected with hormones** or fed with commercial feed containing any drugs or toxins.

- **Canned soups** – read labels for sugar, salt, starch, flour and preservatives.

- **Foods containing preservatives, additives,** benzoate of soda, salt, sugar, cream of tartar, drugs, irradiated and genetically engineered foods.

- **Day-old cooked vegetables,** potatoes and pre-mixed, wilted lifeless salads.

- **All commercial vinegars:** pasteurized, filtered, distilled, white, malt and synthetic vinegars are dead vinegars! (We use only unfiltered Apple Cider Vinegar with "Mother Enzyme" as used in olden times.)

Please follow The Bragg Healthy Lifestyle to provide the basic, healthy nourishment to maintain your precious health.

Step 2: Analyze Your Own Health

The next thing to do before you go on The Bragg Healthy Lifestyle is to sit down and carefully analyze yourself! You know how you feel. No one in the world could diagnose in detail your problems. Therefore you must do some wise self-diagnosing, keep a daily journal – page 74. Now re-read list of clogging, toxic-forming foods.

So now balance your ailments against your diet – you may have had bronchitis or asthma, etc. for many years – all this must be taken into consideration before you can live completely on The Toxicless Diet, Body Purification and Healing System. You've got to consider if you have had any operations, and how many harmful foods, drinks and drugs you have used! You then not only have to flush out food toxins, but if you have used drugs of any kind, they too may be buried deeply into body tissues and must be flushed out!

Ask yourself these vital questions: How much meat, eggs and dairy products do you eat? These questions will all have to be carefully considered. After you have responsibly analyzed all factors of your diet, food intake, habits, etc., you are ready to move on to the third step.

Free yourself from bondage of these habits:

✦ "I will not use tobacco."   ✦ "I will not over-eat."

✦ "I will not drink coffee, sodas and alcoholic drinks."

✦ "I will not clog my arteries with saturated fats."

The unexamined life is not worth living. It is a time to re-evaluate your past as a guide for a bright, healthy future.
– Socrates, ancient Greek Philosopher

Who is strong? He that can conquer his bad habits.
– Benjamin Franklin

Those who persevere through hard times will reap great rewards when the tide turns . . . and the tide always turns." – Joe Mitchell, American writer best known for work published in "The New Yorker"

Seek and find the best for your body, mind and soul. – Patricia Bragg

Step 3: Your Individual Transition Diet

We want you to remember first, and bear in mind at all times, that **the ideal diet of man is raw and lightly cooked fruits; raw, steamed or baked vegetables, brown rice, beans, legumes, raw nuts and seeds.** Include a healthy abundance of raw and lightly cooked green-leafed vegetables, such as chard, spinach, beet tops, mustard and turnip greens, broccoli, collards and kale. Please be ambitious in following this Bragg Lifestyle with internal cleansing, so to reach the ideal state of purification. There are various degrees of health that can be obtained by controlling the diet. We feel that if a person can reach the point where their diet contains from 60% -70% organic raw fruits and vegetables – with a minimum amount of protein, fats and sugars – they can live in a higher state of health for a long, vigorous life. (*See Healthy Plant Based Daily Food Guide on page 51.*)

The Transition Diet starts first with a distilled water (or juice) fast for 24 hours (see pages 133, 138-139). Fasting is a miracle detoxifier because, when we stop eating, all of our Vital Force which was used to masticate, digest and assimilate food and eliminate waste is now used to purify the body! All this energy is then used to release and flush out accumulated obstructions and stored toxic poisons from the body! (Read our book *The Miracle of Fasting.*) After each 24 hour fast make it an iron-firm rule always to begin every meal with something raw. This will re-educate the 260 taste buds of your mouth to the delicate natural flavors of raw foods. This can't be accomplished if a person smokes cigarettes, cigars or a pipe, because taste and flavors are wasted completely on a smoker and also on alcohol, coffee, and cola drinkers!

Please eliminate smoking, alcohol, salt and all unhealthy beverages (including coffee, soda and sugary juices) from your diet. Table salt (*from land and sea sources*) is best eliminated, (Celtic Salt allowed if desired). We use no table salt (*inorganic sodium*) in or on our foods! You get ample organic sodium found naturally in foods. To add delicious, healthier flavors to foods use onions, garlic, coconut aminos and fresh herbs including sea kelp!

Step 4: Be Ready for Your Healing Crisis

The healing crisis is one of the great mysteries of The Toxicless Diet, Body Purification and Healing System. Most humans have been so indoctrinated with the idea that when you have something wrong with you and you want to improve your health, you get a physical examination. You are then "diagnosed" and a name is given to your ailment. Treatment is begun and you believe that you are going to feel better, stronger and will soon "get well." Don't expect to feel this way on The Toxicless Diet, Body Purification and Healing System! As you start on this System of Purification you are going to stir up old toxic poisons, and you do have plenty of them! Everyone else also has them, because almost everyone carries from 5-10 pounds of deeply buried toxic poisons in their bodies at all times.

That's what sickness is in the final true analysis – the body becomes so corroded and loaded with vicious toxic poisons that it throws up its own cleansing purge or healing crisis. This healing crisis is the body's urgent response to the need to get clean and healthy! This cleansing can take the form of a cold, flu, pneumonia, fevers, headaches, coughs, earaches, boils, skin eruptions abscesses and hundreds of other manifestations of the body ridding itself of toxic poisons. Disease is no mystery to us! These toxins do not come like a thief in the night, but are slowly created by an unhealthy diet and lifestyle habits, eventually leading to the accumulation of deadly toxins in the pipe system and every organ of the body.

We are not going to tell you that when you go on the Transition Diet – along with your 24 hour weekly fast, combined with eating more organic fruits and vegetables and eliminating some of the heavier foods – that you are going to feel good right away. You may not feel your best until you have eliminated a large amount of the hidden toxic poisons from your body. It takes time.

We don't give special diets for special ailments. We believe in living a 100% healthy lifestyle. You must slowly, through water fasting and eating more raw organic fruits and vegetables, help your body detox and flush out the heavy toxic poisons that have built up over the years!

Step 5: Enjoy The Universe's Health Benefits

Our bodies are miracle instruments. The cleaner they become through The Toxicless Diet, Body Purification and Healing System, the more oxygen they will absorb, which is the source of all life. A toxin-polluted body can only take in so much oxygen when it is encumbered with so many obstructions! As you purify your body, it will feast on the invisible foods of the universe! Your body will absorb more oxygen, more energy, more ozone and more of the sun's strength-giving, gentle rays. Think of it – living on the invisible foods of Mother Nature! Babies do this – they eat only a small amount of food, and mother's milk is only 3.5% protein. Have you ever watched a healthy, active baby kick and wiggle and coo for hours at a time? Where is the energy coming from? Not from the mother's milk with only 3.5% protein! That baby's body is clean because of the powerful, invisible nutrients gathered from the Universe. Look at the baby's delicate skin, see his wide, bright eyes, sunny smile and listen to his powerful lungs support his cries when he wants something or he's wet!

If we could only burn into your consciousness the one simple fact that toxic wastes are poisonous agents that deteriorate and slowly kill human flesh, then half of our Crusade work is accomplished! Naturally an adult that lives an active life in the sun and the fresh air is going to have a more mature skin than a 5-month-old baby, but that doesn't mean it must appear to be an old skin! We have seen men and women in their 80s, 90s and older who barely had a wrinkle or line on their face. Dr. John Harvey Kellogg was one of the greatest American Health Doctors who ever lived. The last time my father saw him, the famous doctor was giving a health lecture in his nineties! He had the skin of a young man and a smooth face that literally shined with health like a polished apple! **This is what my father and I wish for you, our new health friend and reader – a body glowing with super, optimum health for a long, happy life!**

What wound did ever heal but by gentle degrees? – William Shakespeare

Step 6: "No Heavy Breakfast" Plan is Best

Our combined experience of over 150 years has proven to us that a carefully selected and progressively changed Transition Diet is the best way for every person to obtain their fulfilling goal of Total Health. But when people still live on unhealthy, refined foods, they must not eat too many fresh fruits and vegetables at first. Also every person must learn, if they truly want to attain perfection, they should not eat a heavy morning breakfast that saps their energy! We have seen people banish physical problems after going on the "no heavy breakfast" plan, combined with a healthy diet with plenty of fresh organic fruits and vegetables and fresh juices and some faithful fasting!

When you give up breakfast you will be thrilled and have all the more Super Energy to enjoy! In our personal lives, my father and I did most of our creative work in the morning. And when it was time for our daily physical activity – such as hiking, swimming, tennis or other sports – we were still filled with vital strength. Remember, it takes tremendous energy to digest a heavy breakfast! You can't put your energy in two arenas at once, into both food and activity. People wonder why we accomplished so much between 6 a.m. and noon. It was because we didn't dissipate our Vital Force on a big breakfast! **Our daily Apple Cider Vinegar Drink, whole or juiced fruit or Bragg Energy Smoothie (page 71) is all we need – and we have inexhaustible super energy!**

You will continually hear people say, "Breakfast is the most important meal of the day." This is simply not true! Scientifically, it takes a tremendous amount of nervous energy to chew, digest, absorb and eliminate a typical American breakfast! The average person believes that a hearty breakfast is going to give them strength. They believe this having been brainwashed by TV and print commercials and propaganda created for the producers of modern breakfast products: cereals, breads, pancakes, waffles, eggs, sausage, bacon, tea, coffee, cocoa, milk, etc. It's in their financial interest to have people believing they need a big breakfast for lots of energy.

24

Let's look at it from a Scientific viewpoint. If you eat a breakfast of cereal or hot cakes with 2 eggs, bacon, 3 slices of buttered toast and a beverage like tea or coffee, it is not immediately converted into energy! You must realize it takes a great deal of time and energy for your stomach to mix this unnecessary, heavy breakfast with the digestive juices for the slow process of digestion and assimilation. Then the separation process takes place as proteins are broken down by special juices in the stomach and fats, starches and sugars are pushed into the small intestine for later digestion. After the food has been broken down into a fine liquid by the digestive tract, it still hasn't been absorbed by the body. The liquefied food then must move past little tissues known as "villi" that line the intestines. The suckers of the tiny villi then draw nourishment into your blood.

Again, we must emphasize that this entire process takes hours – so if anyone says that you get immediate strength from eating a heavy breakfast, you know they are totally ignorant of the facts of digestion! You may say, "Yes, that's very well but I'm hungry in the morning. I get up hungry!" We will have to answer that you are all wrong – your stomach has been conditioned to load up with food in the morning. What you mistake for hunger is simply a reflex action enforced by a long-term habit of eating a big, heavy breakfast! Once you discard breakfast and begin to live on the "no heavy breakfast" plan, you will never again put a heavy amount of food into your stomach in the morning. **A heavy breakfast makes you sluggish and sleepy just when you need go-power to start your day!**

Don't Let Johnny Appleseed's Dream Die!

The legendary "Johnny Appleseed – the apple tree angel" wandered the wilds of Eastern America in the early 1800's planting apple trees. Over 200 years later some of those trees are still bearing fruit. But in today's world large seed companies are striving to make what Johnny Appleseed did illegal. Giant companies like Monsanto, are striving to stop farmers worldwide from saving and reusing their seeds from year to year. We must protest against Monsanto's efforts to control the world's seeds! Please call or e-mail the President, your Governor, Senators, and state officials at: usa.gov. Visit website: Mercola.com

You have just begun to reap the many rewards of The Bragg Healthy Lifestyle! First you eliminated your body's toxic poisons. Soon your aches, pains and physical miseries will start to vanish! Then your energy is lifted to a higher degree and you no longer suffer from excessive fatigue! Yes, these changes will be life-changing and miraculous! Life is precious and you will be proud of the health improvements you are making! **You are now taking responsibility for your own health and fitness as the Captain of Your Life by steering towards super health, happiness and longevity!**

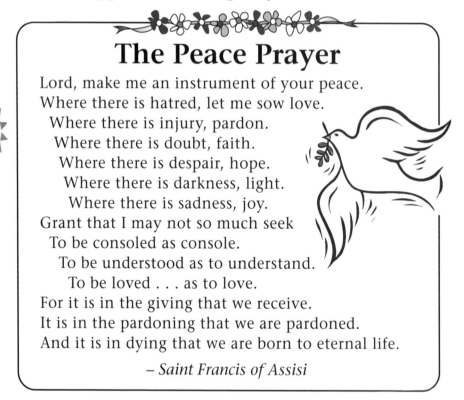

The Peace Prayer

Lord, make me an instrument of your peace.
Where there is hatred, let me sow love.
Where there is injury, pardon.
Where there is doubt, faith.
Where there is despair, hope.
Where there is darkness, light.
Where there is sadness, joy.
Grant that I may not so much seek
To be consoled as console.
To be understood as to understand.
To be loved . . . as to love.
For it is in the giving that we receive.
It is in the pardoning that we are pardoned.
And it is in dying that we are born to eternal life.

– Saint Francis of Assisi

26

There is only one corner of the universe that you can be certain of improving and that's your own self. – Aldous Huxley

Living in harmony with the Universe is living totally alive, full of vitality, health, joy, power, love, and abundance on every level. – Shakti Gawain

God will not change the condition of men, until they change what is in themselves. – Quran, classic Arabic literature and sacred texts

Chapter 3

Vitality From The Universe

Remain Active, Youthful, Healthy and Graceful

In our professional life as Pioneer Health and Fitness Advisors to the Film Stars of Hollywood, we have had many female clients who absolutely defied time! They reaped the benefits of The Bragg Healthy Lifestyle – The Toxicless Diet, Body Purification and Healing System. You could never quite determine their age because at 50 they looked 30, while at 60 they looked and acted like only 40! This is what we want for both women and men; to look, feel and act years younger and have zest and go-power for a healthy, happy, long fulfilled life!

The outward signs of this age-defying youthfulness are a straight-back and a handsome posture, supple breast contours, healthy smooth skin on face and neck, firm muscles and that particular vigorous grace typical of an active, healthy female. At age 50, 65, 75, and more these women still look quite attractive and youthful.

To the emotionally mature woman, this physical attractiveness is rarely an end in itself; rather, it's a subtle means by which she relates to the world around her. This quality derives its charm from her balanced physical, emotional, spiritual and mental self-confidence.

Women Be Ageless and Youthful – Why Not?

Now, thanks to The Bragg Toxicless Diet, Body Purification and Healing System, it is possible for a woman to retain her vitality – as well as her physical and sexual appeal – throughout her long, healthy life! By retaining these attributes, she also safeguards a less direct, more elusive aspect of her total feminine personality. **We believe women can remain active, youthful, healthy, graceful and strong for their entire long life!** Loss of vitality can be a thing of the past for any woman who will invest her time and has the discipline to guide her body by living The Bragg Healthy Lifestyle!

Most Men Sadly Today Are Health Sinners!

Men, we're not forgetting you, this applies to all of you too! We know that women typically take better care of themselves. Many men destroy themselves with tobacco, alcohol and a heavy meat, fat and sugar diet. It's a well-known fact women live anywhere from 5 to 10 years longer than the average man! For most men a couple of beers and a pizza or a big steak and a large pile of fried potatoes is good eating. That's one reason that men are dying off prematurely in alarming numbers! Our civilized world is full of widows simply because a large majority of men are ignorant about the importance of a healthy lifestyle! Men ridicule the very idea of good nutrition, and reject the value of eating fresh organic fruits, fresh juices, vegetables, salads, etc., as well as getting sufficient regular exercise to keep the body's machinery and muscular structure healthy, trim and fit.

28

Not only do many men die young but, either through ignorance or willfulness, they will not follow the basic principles of natural nutrition and soon suffer from many physical ailments! The average man of 40 in most countries today is a candidate for a heart attack or some other chronic disease and an early death! Most men living on this heavy, meat-toxic diet lose their Adam Power very early in life! Our civilized world has men in their 30s, 40s, and 50s complaining of being totally impotent! Many of these men suffer from a diseased, enlarged prostate.

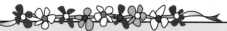

The Body is Self-Cleansing, Self-Healing and Self-Repairing

It's our duty if we want vibrant, glorious health, to do all we can to make the body work efficiently to maintain vital, super health. Not only is a healthy diet necessary, but so are good sleeping habits, outdoor physical activity, full, deep breathing and a serene, peaceful mind! We cannot live by bread alone. We must have spiritual food. Please strive for a perfect healthy balance: physical, mental, emotional and spiritual well-being!

Healthy, healing dietary fibers are organic fresh vegetables, fruits, salads whole grains and their products. These health builders help normalize your blood pressure, cholesterol and promotes healthy elimination.

Self discipline is your golden key; without it, you cannot be happy.
– Maxwell Maltz, M.D., author "Cybernetics"

Toxic Poisons Cause Hormone Imbalance!

No wonder divorce rates of "civilized" countries are staggering. When toxic poisons get into the reproductive glands of both male and female, serious problems arise! Sexual desires diminish as more toxic chemicals build up in the body's delicate organs.

There is no biological reason why men and women cannot retain their sexual energies up to 90 and longer! There is a great deal of proof in the world that this is true. One need only to look at the children that actors Charlie Chaplin and Tony Randall and artist Pablo Picasso fathered in their 70s and 80s for proof of the human machine's incredible, long-lasting fertility! In fact, a male's fertility can last an entire lifetime! The only thing that can happen to the reproductive organs of both the male and female is a diseased condition caused by an unfortunate incident, accident or the individual's ignorance of the importance of living a healthy lifestyle.

Yet we have had men in the TV and film industry who, through following our advice, had been able to retain their strong bodies. They also had youthful voices even though they were in their 50s, 60s, 70s, 80s and more. They felt and acted at least 20-30 years younger than their actual age! Also, we have consulted with top business men who are now in their 60s and 70s, looked only 30 or 40! Why stop wanting to look younger? Start living The Bragg Healthy Lifestyle to look, feel and act years younger! Conrad Hilton added more years to his life! It's never too late to make healthy changes in your lifestyle!

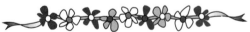

I have the wisdom of my years and the youthfulness of The Bragg Healthy Lifestyle and I never act or feel my calendar years! I feel ageless! Why shouldn't you? Start living the Bragg Healthy Way today!
– Patricia Bragg

Man is fully responsible for his nature and his choices. – Jean-Paul Sartre

Nutrition directly affects growth, development, reproduction and health of an individual's physical and mental condition. Health depends upon nutrition and is the most important factor!
– Dr. W. H. Sebrell, Jr., Nutrition Expert and Pioneer in Vitamin Research

Conrad Hilton Thanks Bragg for His Long Life!

When the world's biggest hotel magnate Conrad Hilton was all of 80 and lying on his deathbed, we gave him a new lease on life by introducing him to The Bragg Healthy Lifestyle. He followed our instructions and discovered a whole new healthy, vibrant lifestyle! He was soon healthy, happy and fit, enjoying life! He even remarried at 88 years young! He remained active in business (half days at his office) and lived happily into his 90's! Mr. Hilton at 88 was quoted in a *People Magazine* interview as saying, *"I wouldn't be alive today if it wasn't for the Braggs and their Bragg Healthy Lifestyle!"* With this magazine article was a photo of the grateful hotel millionaire with his healthy lifestyle teacher, Patricia Bragg.

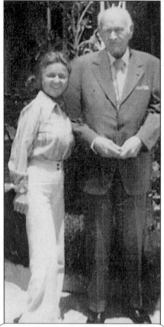

Patricia with Conrad Hilton

30

Eternally Youthful – Bob Cummings

Bob Cummings was one of Broadway and Hollywood's talented early successes, who also pioneered TV with his wholesome family series "My Little Margie." Bob followed The Bragg Healthy Lifestyle from 18 when he was the toast of Broadway. Bob C. was the singing and dancing Star of Ziegfeld's Folly *"A Pretty Girl Is Like a Melody."* At his mother's insistence, Bob attended a Bragg Health Crusade in New York City's Times Square on his night off. It changed his life! **My father's message penetrated Bob's heart, soul and mind, inspiring him to become a faithful Bragg follower. We are proud to note that when Bob reached his 70s, he still retained the youthful energy and posture of a man in his 30s!** *You can too!*

What you focus on – you manifest in your life!

LaLanne Thanks Bragg for Healthy, Long Life!

Another success story and example of how attending one of our Bragg Health Crusade lectures can change someone's life with total health is found in a once-sickly 15-year old, now famous for the 35-year run of his TV *Jack LaLanne Exercise Show!* Over 80 years ago Jack's mother dragged her ailing son to a lecture being given by my Health Crusading father. They arrived late, the hall was packed, and they had to sit on the stage close to Paul lecturing in front of 3,000 people. Jack LaLanne said:

"I had dropped out of school for over a year. I was a shut-in! I had pimples and boils, and wore glasses. I was thin and so weak I had to wear a back brace and couldn't participate in sports. I didn't want anyone to see me. I was weak and sick. I used to have blinding headaches every day and I couldn't stand the pain. I wanted to get out of this body I had. Paul Bragg told me I could be born again and be healthy, strong and fit if I changed to The Bragg Healthy Lifestyle! He asked me, 'What do you eat for breakfast, lunch and dinner?' And I told him, 'Cakes, pies, ice cream, and candy!' He said, 'Jack, you are a walking garbage can.' That night I got down on my knees, by the side of my bed, and prayed. I didn't say, 'God, make me a Mr. America.' I said, 'God, please give me the will-power and intestinal fortitude to refrain from eating unhealthy, lifeless foods when the urge comes over me. Please give me strength to exercise when I don't feel like it.' **God was good and inspired me to be strong and healthy!"**

An Old English Prayer

Give us Lord, a bit o' sun,
A bit o' work and a bit o' fun.
Give us in all the struggle and sputter,
Our daily bread and a bit of butter.
Give us health, our keep to make
And a bit to spare for others' sake.
Give us too, a bit of song,
And a tale and a book, to help us along.
Give us Lord, a chance to be
Our goodly best, brave, wise and free.
Our goodly best for ourselves and others,
'Til all men learn to live as brothers.

Jack LaLanne Became Healthy, Youthful And Ageless – You Can Be Too!!!

There wasn't a jelly donut in Jack's life since! Jack LaLanne faithfully followed The Bragg Healthy Lifestyle since that night. Jack spread the gospel of health and exercise through his great TV shows and website that had all the past history of his

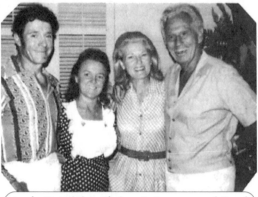

Jack, Patricia, Elaine LaLanne and Paul

long successful life to 97½ years. This happily married father of two celebrated on his 70th birthday with a mile-long swim towing 70 rowboats carrying 70 people to show his super strength! Jack LaLanne remained strong, healthy and youthful during his long fulfilled life, helping millions to health and fitness!

Jack says, "Bragg saved my life at age 15, when I attended the Bragg Health Crusade in Oakland, California." From that day on, Jack continued to live The Bragg Healthy Lifestyle, inspiring millions to health and fitness with his TV show! Please visit web: JackLaLanne.com

"Gardenburger" Creator Thanks Bragg Books

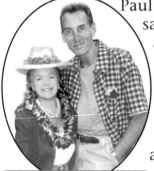

Patricia with Paul Wenner

Paul Wenner, the Gardenburger Creator, says his early years as a youth with asthma were so bad he would stand at the window praying to breathe through the night and stay alive. A miracle happened when as a teenager he read the Bragg Books *The Miracle of Fasting* and *Bragg Healthy Lifestyle* and his years of asthma were cured in only one month. Paul became so inspired that he wanted to be a Health Crusader like Paul Bragg and his daughter Patricia – and Paul Wenner did! Gardenburgers were sold worldwide and were one of the first meatless burgers! *GardenBurger.com*

"Good Earth" Founder Thanks Bragg Books

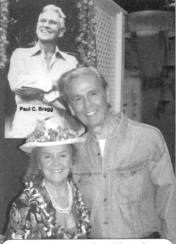

Paul C. Bragg

Bill Galt, the founder of The Good Earth Restaurant chain, charged himself with Super Health and changed his entire life after reading Bragg books *The Miracle of Fasting* and *Bragg Vegetarian Health Recipes*. His entire family followed The Bragg Healthy Lifestyle. Their friends and associates wanted to know what was the cause of the miraculous changes they

Patricia with Bill Galt & Paul Bragg's Picture

saw in the Galts! Their friends wanted what they had – Super Health! Bill and his family started a tiny restaurant that served only lunches. An overnight success, they started serving a full vegetarian menu all day. Soon they expanded and opened a chain of health restaurants, all serving delicious healthy food based on The Bragg Healthy Lifestyle! We were blessed to have a Good Earth Restaurant in Santa Barbara. Many Hollywood Stars often ate there, including Jack LaLanne.

33

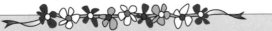

Dr. Paul C. Bragg says . . . "Life is Thrilling When You Can Help Others!" Bragg Stay Ageless Program promotes lifelong health and fitness through the simple Bragg Healthy Lifestyle! Remember – we are linked to Mother Earth through the food we eat, water we drink, air we breathe, thoughts we think, things we do and the sun with its life-giving power. God has truly blessed me! Start living The Bragg Healthy Lifestyle today!

Many people go through life committing partial suicide – destroying their health, youth, energy and creativity. Indeed, to learn how to be good to oneself is often more difficult than to learn how to be good to others. – Dr. Paul C. Bragg

The chemistry of food a person eats becomes his own body chemistry. Perhaps the most valuable result of all education is the ability to inspire and make yourself do the thing you have to do, when it ought to be done, as it ought to be done, whether you like to do it or not! – Patricia Bragg, Pioneer Health Crusader

You Can Create New Health and Vitality!

When you faithfully follow The Bragg Toxicless Diet, Body Purification and Healing System, you will feel and see startling body changes in the mirror. When you start the elimination process, occasionally you will look tired. This sometimes happens during a cleansing-healing crisis, when the greatest amount of toxic poisons are being flushed out of the pipes and vital organs of the body. After you have gone through several cleansing-healing crises you can then see the New, Healthier You revealing itself! Your eyes become brighter, your skin and muscle tone healthier and the joints of your body more supple. **Your entire body throbs with a state of well-being that makes you glad to be alive!**

Each day when you live on The Toxicless Diet, Body Purification and Healing System you make changes and adjustments that help create a new, stronger, more vigorous and healthy body! To my father and me it's worth all the effort and dedication that goes into living this healthy lifestyle. Man has strayed from it because of the pressures of our modern, highly commercial world. If he is to survive in this world, man must change his life over to a healthier, peaceful lifestyle!

The degree of physical perfection you wish to attain is solely a personal matter and up to you! You must remember that 60 to 70% of your diet should consist of raw organic fruits, vegetables, sprouts and fresh juices. Your vegetarian protein, plus natural sugars, oils, starches and carbohydrates will make up the balance, pages 52-54.

We must remind you that we offer no special diets for any specific ailments! We recognize only one cause for all ailments – internal toxic clogging! When you loosen and flush these vicious obstructions from your body, then you are taking The Bragg Royal Road to Total Health!

You can be a sewage system when eating unhealthy, highly processed foods. Remember, live foods produce healthy, living, live people!

Progress is impossible without change, and those who cannot change their minds, cannot change anything. – George Bernard Shaw

Please Have Patience – It Takes Time and Dedication To Reach Internal Perfection!

Constantly keep in mind that it took you years to get in the condition you are now. Now you must be patient with yourself and Mother Nature and your body. Do not throw caution to the wind! If you have been eating meat several times daily, or eggs and cheese every day, you must slowly eliminate excessive use of these clogging foods. Soon your body won't even miss them!

As you continue your fasting program, plus adding more fresh, raw fruits and vegetables to your diet, you will gradually reach a perfect health balance! This is the stage where toxic poisons are no longer retained in the body and it becomes mucus-free and toxin-free. This means you have reached a peak of internal fitness, a point of perfection! This is the condition everyone should seek! This is what we want for you, our new health friends and readers: to live a long, vibrant, healthy lifestyle and enjoy eating a healthy, balanced diet while maintaining a clean, painless, tireless and ageless body!

Caution – Move Slowly and Patiently For Super Healthy Success in Your Life!

Keep in mind that "the wheels of time move slowly, but surely." You can't rush your body or Mother Nature! You can't be impatient and expect to reach perfect internal fitness in a few months! Rome wasn't built in a day! Achieving Super Health takes both dedication and time!

It is the Body – Not Medicine – That's The Hero!

"It is the body that is the hero, not science, not antibiotics . . . not machines, drugs or new devices. The task of the physician today is what it has always been, to help the body do what it has learned so well to do on its own during its unending struggle for survival to heal itself!"
– Ronald Glasser, M.D., author, *The Body is The Hero*

It's supposed to be a professional secret, but I'll tell you anyway. We doctors do nothing. We only help and encourage the doctor within.
– Albert Schweitzer, Nobel Peace Prize

Age does not depend upon years, but upon lifestyle and health!

You Can Reach Mental and Spiritual Heights You Never Dreamed of

Man is a trinity comprised of the Physical, Mental and the Spiritual. It is difficult trying to reach the heights in the mental and spiritual life when the physical body is decaying. The ancient Greeks envisioned man in perfection as having a strong mind in a strong body!

Today millions of people pray and benefit from a higher spiritual level. They are truth seekers and are reaching out for a better way of life. Before you can become an advanced student in any spiritual and mental philosophy, your body must be clean and free of deadly toxic poisons.

The great spiritual teachers and philosophers have recognized for over 7,000 years the miraculous cleansing power of fasting. Throughout the Bible, Jesus showed us the importance of fasting and prayer for those seeking a closer spiritual walk with God! Buddha, Mohammed, Gandhi, the Popes and many other Spiritual Leaders have recognized fasting as the path to higher spiritual, mental and physical advancements!!

36

Paul C. Bragg's Deep Spiritual Awakening

When I went into this profession years ago my main goal was to be well and stay well. I always wanted to be healthy regardless of calendar years! In other words, I wanted a radiantly healthy body with plenty of strength, endurance, vitality and energy to spare for a long, happy, fulfilled life. I wanted to Crusade and share these health truths with the world! As I attained these goals I realized that The Toxicless Diet, Body Purification and Healing System was opening other channels of thought to me. I found myself searching for simple spiritual truth. My mental energy was so high that I was able to do enormous amounts of reading and studying.

When you begin to believe that you can be what your vision tells you that you can become, that's when your are inspired!

Where there's great love of God and Mother Nature there are always miracles. – Willa Cather, 1873-1947

I sought out brilliant teachers in religion and before I knew it, I was attaining this heavenly serenity and a peace of mind I had never before experienced! My whole personality was changing! I no longer worried and fretted over problems.

In fact, I liked the challenges that difficulties presented. Because I now had, with prayer and my strong spiritual and mental capacity, a way to look objectively at them and find the proper solutions. ***My life was being guided and blessed!***

Our Creator Teaches You to Be A Good Steward of Your Life, Health, Home, Assets and Family

I found myself a happier person. I found little things could make me laugh and fill me with joy. I discovered the beauty of stars at night and the sky during the day. I enjoyed the rain, the wind and I soon became one with Mother Nature! Since my childhood I had carried some fears and anxieties which I now found were not true problems – they faded as the night fades in early morning dawn! I was led from darkness into light, from the unreal to the real. With my fears and anxieties out of my life and consciousness I was ready to follow my dream and passion of being a World Health Crusader. I had no fears of traveling any place in the world and delivering The Bragg Health Crusade. I found I made friends everywhere I lectured. ***I owe this spiritual and mental growth to my healthy lifestyle, prayer time and my walk with God. I learned to concentrate in prayer and quiet time to anticipate future conditions that I must face.***

Learning is finding out what you already knew.
Doing is demonstrating that you know it!
Teaching is reminding others that they know it
just as well as you! You are all learners,
doers and teachers! – Richard Bach

God has a more acceptable plan. He has a plan to bless you,
a plan to heal you, and a plan to protect you!

True wisdom consists in not departing from nature,
but molding our conduct according to her wise laws.
– Seneca, Roman Philosopher and Emperor Nero's Advisor, 65 A.D.

Paul C. Bragg Found Peace, Relaxation and Joy – and then Crusaded to Share it with the World!

Many people talk about relaxing – just as I used to talk about it but only after years of consistent healthy lifestyle with fasting and purification that I really learned to completely relax! Each day I'm able to release all tensions from my nerves and muscles and thus renew my vitality and energy through complete relaxation. I sleep better now than I did when I was a child! I find that no matter where I am – no matter what the noise or excitement may be – I can sit or lie down, close my eyes and completely relax. This I want for you also!

I find I'm able to understand other people now when they become upset and emotional. I'm therefore better able to help them calm down. I feel I'm growing – and not only on the physical side! I believe I'm not only building a powerful physical body but, through Cleansing and Fasting, I'm also advancing Mentally and Spiritually. I constantly search for light, truth and education along all lines. I find I have a greater interest in everything that is happening in the world. I find I understand people better and in understanding others, I'm able to better understand myself. This way of life opens many doors that lead to Higher Life! After all, as we journey through life we should grow and balance our lives Physically, Mentally, Emotionally and Spiritually. Many of our worldwide health followers write us about this newly discovered strength in Mental and Spiritual growth they are experiencing. They rejoice when they have found Peace in their mind, soul and total being. **This is the true Joy of Healthy Living!**

I'm a happy man! I have no worries, no fears and no false ambitions! I lead a simple, healthy, happy fulfilled life and give thanks for all my blessings daily!
Remember Patricia and I are your health friends for eternity.

with love,

Paul C. Bragg

Dear friend, I wish above all things that thou may prosper and be in health even as the soul prospers. – 3 John 2

Nothing in all creation is so like God as soothing stillness. – Meister Eckhart

Chapter 4

Sharing the Principles of The Bragg Healthy Lifestyle

You're on Your Way to Miracle Blessings!

We want you to thoroughly understand that The Toxicless Diet, Body Purification and Healing System is not made up of special diets for specific ailments. There are no special diets given. It is based on the simple principle that the body will naturally heal and maintain itself after the individual begins to follow The Bragg Healthy Lifestyle which eliminates the deeply buried toxic poisons, obstructions and encumbrances that have been accumulating in the body for years. If any drugs have been taken, residue of these chemicals will still be buried deep in the spongy organs and tissues of the body and must also be removed before they cause trouble.

39

During his early years Paul suffered from TB as a teenager and was given enormous amounts of powerful drugs. It took him many years to eliminate those drugs from his tissues through fasting and living closely to Mother Nature! He went through a number of healing crises in those years before he was totally free from the vicious drugs given to him. Read our book *The Miracle of Fasting* (see pages 175-178). It's inspired millions, even in Russia to live a Healthy Lifestyle – it's been the #1 health book in Russia for over 40 years. This life-changing book has altered the lives of millions worldwide – from The Beach Boys, who over 40 years ago used our teachings to get off drugs and alcohol, to Dick Gregory, who went from an unhealthy 350 pounds to a trim, fit, healthy 150 pounds. Dick even ran in 8 Boston Marathons!

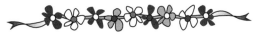

Good health and good sense are two of life's greatest blessings.
– Publilius Syrus, Latin writer, 42 B.C.

Laws of Nature are just, and can be harsh! There's no weak mercy in them. Cause and consequence are inseparable and inevitable!
– Henry Wadsworth Longfellow, an American poet, 1807-1882

The Toxicless Diet, Body Purification and Healing System goes directly to the root cause of your physical problems. The System has no interest in the symptomatic effect of an individual's ailments. Sadly, most people just overlook warnings, rather than deal with the root cause of their ills. We believe that most all physical problems are caused by an excessive accumulation of toxic waste and poisons (from unhealthy foods) in the pipes, tissues and organs of the body. We also believe only a combination of a healthy lifestyle with a balanced natural diet and regular fasting program will help flush these long-buried toxic poisons out of the body. Read page 137 "The Joys of Fasting."

Many people blame their physical problems are caused by tension, stresses or emotional upsets. A strong, clean and toxin-free body can beat most all health and nervous problems! Some people will say that all their problems are due to nerves. Healthy nerves that are free of toxic poisons can meet almost any crisis! Read our book *Building Powerful Nerve Force & Positive Energy* (see page 177). Many people with deep-seated physical problems want to blame everything on an outside agent. When you start this program you must first admit that only you are responsible for your physical condition, and that you alone are solely responsible for improving yourself!

Only Mother Nature and You Can Cure You

Some people may have brought on their troubles because they were ignorant of the great Nutritional Laws of Life dictated by Mother Nature (see page 49). Others realize that following The Bragg Healthy Lifestyle is the single most important factor in regaining and maintaining their health! But many will lack the inner strength to battle their false desires for unhealthy, refined, processed, sugared, dead foods and will continue to build up the poisons in their bodies with their unhealthy lifestyles!

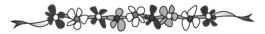

Every man is the builder of a temple called his body. We all are our own sculptors and painters, and our material is our own flesh and blood and bones. Any nobleness begins at once to refine a man's features, any meanness or sensuality to degrade them. – Henry David Thoreau, 1854

Each individual must face the fact that only through their own daily constructive, healthful actions can they heal themselves! This is a cold, hard fact – everything in this life has a price! If you want Higher Supreme Health and wish to extend your life, you must pay the price with dedicated follow through! This means being faithful to your healthy lifestyle and being consistent with your weekly 24-hour cleansing water fast. **We fast every Monday and the first 3 days of every month. Our fast days provide us with more leisure and free time as our body works at "cleaning house!" Try it, you will love it!**

Internal Purity Promotes Youthfulness

The energy and vitality of a young child can be yours at any age when you choose to follow Mother Nature's and God's Eternal Laws of Life. Following this System provides you with the vitality of youth, because youthfulness is Internal Purity! Total Health is not a matter of age, but it's a matter of Internal Perfection!

41

My father in his late seventies was physically younger than a fit man of 40! We do not live by calendar years! We live in biological years and this is what counts! How clean are your arteries and veins? How are your blood pressures? Ours are 120 over 60 like healthy youngsters. We've both had a steady, strong pulse of 60. We've had strong eyes and ears that could hear every sound. We are not interested in birthdays (*forget them*)! We've loved living our Bragg Healthy Lifestyle which has kept us internally cleansed, healthy, ageless, youthful and happy!

You will reap the same benefits my father and I enjoyed when you seriously follow this Toxicless Diet, Body Purification and Healing System! But you must be faithful every day and be the healthy captain of your life! This is not a fad diet – most diets are "yo-yo" diets where your weight just goes up and down! **The Bragg Healthy Lifestyle is something that becomes a part of you and your daily lifestyle and it's not a diet per se – but a lifelong lifestyle for super health and longevity!**

Old age is not a time of life. It is a condition of the body.
It's not time that ages the body, it's abuse that does! – Herbert Shelton

The Bragg Healthy Lifestyle
Promotes Super Health and Longevity

The Bragg Healthy Lifestyle consists of eating a diet of 60% to 70% fresh, live, organically grown foods; raw garden salads, vegetables, fresh fruits and juices; sprouts, raw seeds and nuts; 100% whole-grain breads, pastas, cereals and nutritious beans and legumes. These are the no cholesterol, no fat, no refined salt, "live foods" which combine to make up the body fuel that creates healthy, happy lively people. This is the reason people become revitalized and reborn into a fresh new life filled with joy, health, vitality, youthfulness and longevity! **There are millions of healthy Bragg followers around the world proving that this natural lifestyle works miracles!**

Enjoy a Tireless – Painless – Ageless – Body
Living The Bragg Healthy Lifestyle

42

Most people have a dreadful fear of growing old. They are afraid of becoming a burden to themselves, their family and friends. This is not inevitable!

However, don't despair in your golden years – enjoy them! My father, Paul C. Bragg, said life's second half is the best and can be your most fruitful years! Linus Pauling, Grandma Moses and Mother Teresa have all proven that! Three famous men – Conrad Hilton, JC Penney and foot Doctor Scholl were all Bragg health followers and lived strong, productive, active lives into their 90's. Millions of others worldwide have lived long, healthy lives following The Bragg Healthy Lifestyle.

We teach you how to forget calendar years and to regain not only a youthful spirit, but much of the vigor of your youth. It's your duty to yourself to start to live The Bragg Healthy Lifestyle today – don't procrastinate!

Stop procrastinating for the "right moment" – take action today
- *Read, plan, plot, and follow through for supreme health and longevity.*
- *Underline, highlight or dog-ear pages as you read important passages.*
- *Organizing your lifestyle helps you identify what's important in your life.*
- *Be faithful to your health goals everyday for a healthy, long, happy life.*

Lift up, square your shoulders and look life straight in the face. Keep premature ageing out of your body by following The Bragg Healthy Lifestyle System. You must eat foods that have a high energy life vibration (an abundance of raw, organic fruits and vegetables) and do a water fast one day a week. Exercise and also do Bragg Super Power Deep Breathing. Get 8 hours of restful sleep at night and keep your body relaxed. Don't let anything rob you of your emotional and nervous energy and precious Vital Force. Do read our *Nerve Force* book.

Your body is being made anew every day! Premature ageing and senility result from toxic debris buildup that accumulates when you live an unhealthy lifestyle. Eat right, exercise for good circulation throughout your body, and there will be little or no buildup of toxins that will clog up and prematurely age your body!

Cultivate and hold onto the spirit of youth and it will be yours! You can feel younger! You can look younger! Keep your spine straight to maintain high energy level. Do The Bragg Posture Exercise (page 89) and **follow The Bragg Healthy Lifestyle daily and you'll see miracles!**

If you find you're already in the clutches of premature ageing, begin your fight for the return of youthfulness. Start your Health Crusade today to revitalize your priceless body and health! We have faith you can!

Train your body as an athlete would. Follow our clear, concise instructions and soon you will regain strength, virility, energy, vivacity and enthusiasm! Enjoy that most precious of all earthly gifts – the power and joys of youthful, healthful living. Men and women can become more youthful no matter what their age! Go for it! You can retain the spirit of youth beyond the century mark!

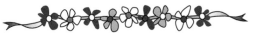

Health is the most natural thing in the world. It is natural to be healthy because we are a part of Mother Nature – we are nature. Nature is trying hard to keep us well, because she needs us in her business. – Elbert G. Hubbard, American writer, artist and philosopher, 1856-1915

The body and mind are so closely connected that not even a single word or thought can come into existence without being reflected in the personality & health of the individual. – John Holmes Prentiss, 1784-1861

Start Your Detox – How To Flush Toxic Poisons Out of Your Body!

1. **Eliminate all toxic foods from your diet forever!** See **Step** 1 (page 18) and page 19 for *Foods To Avoid* list.

2. **Complete a water-only 24-hour fast every 7 days.** See **Step** 3 (page 21). Our book *The Miracle of Fasting* has more information you need to know on this life-saving subject. You will extend your life, plus save 15% off your annual food bill! Also do read Chapter 11 for more fasting information.

3. **Eliminate Breakfast for more energy and go power!** (**see Step** 6 page 24). If this proves too difficult, have only fruit or vegetable juice and/or fresh organic fruit, perhaps try our Bragg Healthy Energy Smoothie (page 71). Some people are so habit-bound to a big breakfast that it takes a little time to eliminate this heavy unnecessary meal. If you still feel you need more in your stomach in the morning, try a bowl of organic oatmeal, whole grain cereal or a poached egg on whole grain toast. **Always remember a regular heavy breakfast is the most useless and energy-robbing meal of the day!**

   Every morning upon arising have an apple cider vinegar drink (recipe page 71). Mix 1 to 2 tsps of organic raw apple cider vinegar (*with the "Mother"*) with equal amount of raw honey in 8 oz. glass of distilled or purified water (*diabetics omit honey, use herb stevia – see page 65*). Read our book *Apple Cider Vinegar Miracle Health System* (or see page 50) for more insight into this miracle health tonic.

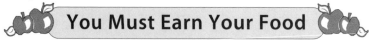
You Must Earn Your Food

4. **By noon you are ready for the first meal of the day.** *You have earned it!* You have used both mental and physical energy. Always start this first important main meal with a large healthy salad (recipe on next page). **Salad is the internal broom. Toxins just have to move out of the body when these live nutrients in raw salads get to work.**

A Large Healthy Salad Recipe . . .

Coarse vegetables – all raw (grate finely if you have chewing problems). Make base of health salad from "Nature's Broom" veggies – chopped or grated cabbage, carrots, beets and celery. To this base add any fresh, raw organic vegetables you desire: cucumbers (with unwaxed skin), lettuce, kale, radishes, parsley, peas, avocado, tomatoes, green onions, mushrooms, red/green bell peppers or any other fresh, raw vegetables. See Bragg Raw Organic Vegetable Health Salad Recipe page 72.

Top this wonderful mixture with fresh salad dressing made of organic raw apple cider vinegar (with the "Mother"), honey and organic extra-virgin olive oil (see page 72). Always eat your fill of raw salad first! Never let hot food touch your mouth until you have finished your health salad!

5. What to eat after your salad only if more is desired? Best would be soup or lightly steamed veggies, greens, carrots, peas, green beans, corn, carrots, beets, broccoli or any vegetables desired and baked potato or whole grain pasta, or lentils and brown rice, tofu, etc. (*recipe page 72*).

Eat Slowly and Chew Thoroughly for Health

If you have not been used to eating large raw vegetable salads, go slowly! Eat slowly and always chew thoroughly. Remember that your stomach has no teeth! You may say, *"Raw salad fills me with gas"* or *"Raw salads do not agree with me."* We can only answer, *"The salads agree with you, but you don't agree with them!"* When a salad does not agree with you, it shows that you have sluggish, unhealthy bowels. In that case there is only one thing to do – gradually change at the speed that fits your condition, also try *Beano.* You can also "eat" your veggies in the form of easily digestible juices. Slowly you will improve to gracefully accept and enjoy these nourishing salads. Remember, salads are the master internal cleansers and "Mother Nature's Broom." (For people with bad dentures or loose teeth, the sick, even toddlers who need nutritious salads, but can't chew well, it's best to finely grate or gently blend salad – it's delicious.)

Everyone is different and this is why you should keep a daily journal (*page 74*) recording your food intake and your reactions for: mucus, headaches, eliminations, energy levels, mood swings, sleep patterns, etc. Start today!

Many times we make a big raw salad for lunch and finish off with some dried fruits such as sun-dried apricots, dates, raisins, figs and some raw nuts.
– Patricia and Paul C. Bragg, N.D., Ph.D., Pioneer Health Crusaders

6. Now we come to the evening meal. There should always be at least 4 to 5 hours between each meal. The digestive system must have time to do its important work efficiently. The evening meal must start with some kind of fresh vegetable salad. If at the noon meal you had a large raw vegetable salad, now you might want a different raw salad. Maybe you would enjoy just a large coleslaw (grated or chopped cabbage) salad; a cabbage, raisin, carrot salad or raw grated beet, cabbage salad. There are many delicious healthy salads a person can select! Check out our salad dressing recipes on page 72. These are easy-to-prepare and delicious, healthy recipes to help you make your meal planning easy and fun!!

You may now have two cooked vegetables – one should be from the yellow variety and the other from the green variety. You could have a dish of lightly steamed or baked carrots and peas or a dish of steamed greens such as chard, kale, spinach, mustard or turnip greens with tomatoes and garlic. These yellow and green vegetables are rich in vital vitamins, minerals and other wonderful nutrients. We prefer you start now to enjoy healthier vegetarian meals. Slowly wean yourself off animal protein and dairy products. Remember protein only in small amounts, see pages 58-60. No one can tell you exactly just how much of these animal foods you can tolerate without problems arising.

46

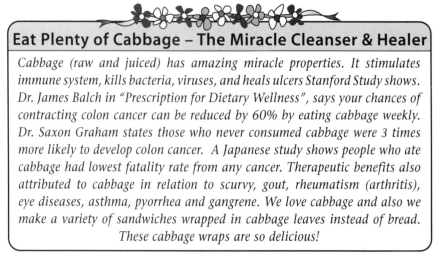

Eat Plenty of Cabbage – The Miracle Cleanser & Healer

Cabbage (raw and juiced) has amazing miracle properties. It stimulates immune system, kills bacteria, viruses, and heals ulcers Stanford Study shows. Dr. James Balch in "Prescription for Dietary Wellness", says your chances of contracting colon cancer can be reduced by 60% by eating cabbage weekly. Dr. Saxon Graham states those who never consumed cabbage were 3 times more likely to develop colon cancer. A Japanese study shows people who ate cabbage had lowest fatality rate from any cancer. Therapeutic benefits also attributed to cabbage in relation to scurvy, gout, rheumatism (arthritis), eye diseases, asthma, pyorrhea and gangrene. We love cabbage and also we make a variety of sandwiches wrapped in cabbage leaves instead of bread.
These cabbage wraps are so delicious!

Animal protein foods (meats, fish, eggs, dairy products) if you want to eat them, should be used with great discretion! It's wise to change over to healthier vegetarian proteins. Personally, we love delicious vegetarian recipes! Try this for 3-4 days and you will soon note the health benefits you feel in your journal (page 74). Forget desserts, only have them once or twice weekly or on special occasions as a treat! If you crave a sweet after a meal, you may have fresh baked apples, stewed fruit or an occasional healthy pie, pastry, cake or cookies made with whole grain flour and honey for dessert. **It's best to avoid daily habit of desserts, however, as it's just another form of overeating! After you have had enough to eat – stop!**

Learn to Simplify and Enjoy Your Meals

Eating should be one of the greatest joys of life! There is a rule we follow in the Bragg home: Always get up from the table feeling you could eat just a little more. Remember that you can also overeat on good, healthy food! The simpler the meal, the better! Most animals live on a mono-diet; that is they eat only one item of food at each meal, and they rarely suffer from the digestive distress man suffers from. **Modern man often desires to overindulge with the six-course dinner or the buffet dinner spread, eating too many mixtures and very often overeating, which only compounds the abuse!**

Go for simplicity in your eating! You will find that the fewer items of food there are at a meal, the less you are tempted to overeat! Make the meal a happy occasion! If it's getting dark, eat by candlelight and play beautiful, soft music. Always take time to chew your food thoroughly and enjoy your healthy meals! Mealtime is no time for serious discussion or arguments! It's a pleasurable, healthy-refueling time in your life!

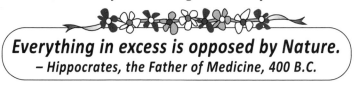

Everything in excess is opposed by Nature.
– Hippocrates, the Father of Medicine, 400 B.C.

No man can violate Nature's Laws and escape her penalties! – Julian Johnson

Healthy, organic foods have an abundance of potential life-giving energy!

Always remember that what you eat and drink today walks and talks tomorrow – it becomes you! You are building yourself with the food you are eating! Give thanks to God and Mother Nature for your meal before you start to eat! It's good for the digestion to be peaceful and say grace! As you eat, millions the world over will go to bed hungry. Malnutrition and starvation are killing millions this very minute, so be thankful for the healthy food you eat! Be thankful you have been led to The Bragg Healthy Lifestyle that will keep you healthier, stronger and more youthful when you wisely follow it faithfully!

Have Special Rejuvenating Health Days

We have "Special Health Days" – on these days we consume only fresh fruit and juice of fresh fruit. Dad and I would often do a few days of only watermelon and its juice when these wonderful melons are blood-red, ripe and plentiful. We called this "The Bragg Watermelon Flush" (great kidney cleanser). We enjoyed going to the beach, lake, river or mountain resort armed with plenty of watermelons, and feasted on absolutely nothing but this fruit for 1-3 days. You may also chew and eat the seeds (helps reduce swelling or edema due to excess retained water from eating processed foods and salt). We loved to cut the watermelon up and make juice, using a juicer or cheesecloth as a strainer. We put this delicious liquid in a glass bottle and refrigerated. When thirsty after hiking, playing tennis, exercising, etc. in the warm sunshine, we would enjoy our watermelon and its juice – you will too!

We often enjoyed days of only fresh, ripe organic fruits, cherries, watermelon, fresh grapes, apricots, etc. (*Save the apricot pits, kernels are high in vitamin B17. Dry, age, and then crack open pits and eat 1-2 kernels a day.*) Very often in our busy lives, we made it strictly a fruit day. We both worked and played harder on our all-fruit detox cleansing day!

When the body is clean and purified you no longer crave rich heavy foods. When you re-educate the 260 taste buds of your mouth, it's almost impossible to let any unhealthy food enter your system. Your clean, newly educated taste buds will refuse to let these foods pass by them. They become the loving, wise guardians of your Holy Temple – Your Body!

Health Miracles Are Within Your Power

Now you have a complete overview of The Toxicless Diet, Body Purification and Healing System: the wise "no heavy breakfast" plan *(only fruit or Healthy Energy Smoothie [children love] page 71)*, water-only fast – one day weekly and slowly add more fresh fruits and raw or lightly cooked vegetables to your diet. When you reach the point where you have fully embraced these principles, the *"New You"* will appear! You'll feel more healthy with more energy, endurance and go-power! You will sleep better and wake well-rested after sleep. Those nagging aches and pains that troubled you will soon fade away. Your eyes will become clearer and skin more youthful. These are the rewards you will receive when following Mother Nature and living by her Wise Laws!

Natural Health Laws for Physical Perfection

These Natural Wise Laws God and Mother Nature put in motion are Perfect Laws created for your own good:

- You must eat natural healthy foods and never overeat

- You must breathe deeply of pure air

- You must exercise the 640 muscles of your body

- You must give your body pure, safe, clean water

- You must give your body gentle sunshine

- You must rest – don't overwork or burden your body;
    this leads to stress and nerve depletion

- You must be clean inside and outside

- You must live by divine intelligence and wisdom

We pray that all our readers will be strong and follow these Natural Health Laws, which are a part of The Bragg Healthy Lifestyle! The human body is a miracle, give it your best! Within us is the inherent potential to become perfect! It's the intent of our Creator for us to have a physically perfect, healthy, happy and peaceful long life! We want you to experience this wonderful health and vitality enjoyed by millions of Bragg followers.

THE MIRACLES OF APPLE CIDER VINEGAR FOR A STRONGER, LONGER, HEALTHIER LIFE

The old adage is true:
"An apple a day keeps the doctor away."

- Helps promote youthful skin and a vibrant healthy body
- Helps remove artery plaque, infections and body toxins
- Helps fight germs, viruses, bacteria and mold naturally
- Helps retard old age onset in humans, pets and farm animals
- Helps regulate calcium metabolism
- Helps keep blood the right consistency
- Helps regulate women's menstruation, relieves PMS, and UTI
- Helps normalize urine pH, relieving frequent urge to urinate
- Helps digestion, assimilation and helps balance the pH
- Helps protect against food poisoning and even brings relief if you do get it
- Helps relieve sore throats, laryngitis and throat tickles and cleans out throat mucus and gum toxins
- Helps detox the body so sinus, asthma and flu sufferers can breathe easier and more normally
- Helps banish acne, athlete's foot, soothes burns, sunburns
- Helps prevent itching scalp, dandruff, and dry hair
- Helps fight arthritis and helps remove crystals and toxins from joints, tissues, organs and entire body
- Helps control and normalize body weight

50

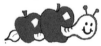

– Paul C. Bragg, N.D., Ph.D., Health Crusader,
Originator of Health Stores

Our sincere blessings to you, dear friends, who make our lives so worthwhile and fulfilled by reading our teachings on natural living as our Creator laid down for us to follow. He wants us to follow the simple path of natural living. This is what we teach in our books and health crusades worldwide. Our prayers reach out to you and your loved ones for the best in health and happiness. We must follow the laws He has laid down for us, so we can reap this precious health physically, mentally, emotionally and spiritually!

HAVE AN APPLE HEALTHY LIFE!   *With Love,*   *Patricia*

Raw organic, unfiltered apple cider vinegar with the "Mother Enzyme" is #1 food I recommend to stop heartburn, gerd, gas, indigestion and for maintaining body's vital acid-alkaline balance and digestion. – Gabriel Cousens, M.D., Author, "Conscious Eating"

Chapter 5

Eat Natural Healthy Foods for Energy & Youthfulness!

Healthy, Organic, High Vibration Foods Contain Life-Giving, Energy Substances

When you eat only foods that are in a high vibration, your body performs and operates by God's Universal Law. It becomes a self-starting, self-cleansing, self-governing, self-generating instrument! **We want you to live by Mother Nature's Laws so your body will be a fine working instrument at every age!**

Start Eating Healthy Foods For Super Energy

The *Healthy Plant-Based Daily Food Guide Pyramid* illustration below, represents an ideal way of eating for achieving optimal nutrition, health and longevity! You will notice that this Food Guide Pyramid is based on healthy organic plant-based foods, with emphasis on

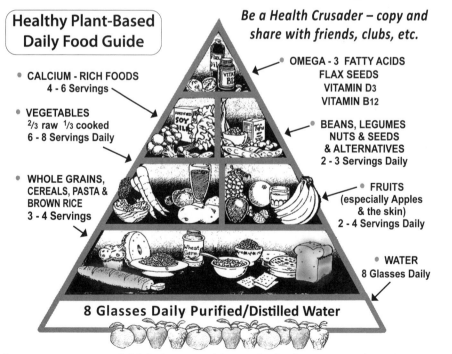

Healthy Plant-Based Daily Food Guide

Be a Health Crusader – copy and share with friends, clubs, etc.

- OMEGA - 3 FATTY ACIDS
  FLAX SEEDS
  VITAMIN D3
  VITAMIN B12

- CALCIUM - RICH FOODS
  4 - 6 Servings

- VEGETABLES
  2/3 raw 1/3 cooked
  6 - 8 Servings Daily

- BEANS, LEGUMES
  NUTS & SEEDS
  & ALTERNATIVES
  2 - 3 Servings Daily

- WHOLE GRAINS,
  CEREALS, PASTA &
  BROWN RICE
  3 - 4 Servings

- FRUITS
  (especially Apples
  & the skin)
  2 - 4 Servings Daily

- WATER
  8 Glasses Daily

8 Glasses Daily Purified/Distilled Water

What a person eats and drinks becomes his own body chemistry. – Dr. Paul C. Bragg

fruits, vegetables, whole grains, vegetable protein foods, non-dairy calcium foods, raw nuts, seeds and purified water. This is the best diet for building a healthy nervous system, disease prevention and to enjoy longevity. *Eating a diet based on these dietary guidelines will help get the nutrients you need for optimal health:*

PURIFIED / DISTILLED WATER: The pyramid's foundation. We recommend drinking distilled water (pages 104-105) it's the best type of water for the body. *Drink at least eight – 8 oz glasses of distilled water daily* and even more if your lifestyle (sports, work, etc.) requires it.

WHOLE GRAINS: Whole grains are next pyramid level. **Avoid GMO process, refined grain products (pages 61-62)** and eat only unrefined, organic whole grain bread and cereals. Grains such as whole wheat, brown rice, oats, millet, quinoa, and 100% whole grain breads and cereals are best. One serving of whole grains is equal to 1 slice whole grain bread, 1 ounce ready-to-eat whole grain cereal, 1 cup cooked whole grains such as brown rice, oatmeal or other grains, 1 cup whole wheat, rice, pasta or noodles, and 1 ounce other whole grain products. *We recommend eating 3-4 servings whole grains a day.* This is because it is challenging to find truly GMO-free wheat in America. Many people of all ages discover they are gluten-sensitive. The wheat of today is not the wheat our grandparents consumed (see pages 61-62). Gluten-free grains such as rice, buckwheat and quinoa are easier to digest and create less mucus as well.

VEGETABLES: We recommend eating as many of your vegetables organic and raw (uncooked, in salads, juices, smoothies, etc.) as possible! When cooking vegetables, do not overcook them. Steaming or lightly stir-frying is best. **The more colorful rainbow of vegetables you eat, the better they are for your health as they contain more valuable nutrients and healthy phytochemicals (page 56).** Eat a wide variety of organic vegetables daily. One vegetable serving is equal to 1 cup cooked vegetables or 1 cup raw uncooked vegetables, 1 cup salad, 3/4 cup vegetable juice. *We recommend 6-8 or more vegetable servings daily.*

Self discipline is your golden key; without it, you can't be happy and healthy.
– Maxwell Maltz, M.D., author, "Psycho-Cybernetics"

FRUITS: Like vegetables, the more colorful the fruits the more healthy for you! Enjoy organic fruits as often as possible! One serving of fruit is equal to 1 medium apple, banana, orange, pear or other fruit, 1/2 cup fruit, 1/2 cup of fruit juice or 1/4 cup dried fruit. *We recommend eating 2-4 servings or more of organic fruits daily.*

CALCIUM FOODS: Are plant-derived calcium-rich foods. Plant sources of calcium are healthier than dairy products because they don't contain saturated fats or cholesterol. Health calcium-rich foods are: soymilk, tofu, broccoli and green leafy vegetables. Serving sizes of plant-derived calcium-rich foods include: 1 cup soymilk, 1/2 cup tofu, 1/3 cup almonds, 1 cup cooked or 2 cups of high calcium raw greens (kale, collards, broccoli, bok choy or other Chinese greens), 1 cup of calcium-rich beans (e.g. soy, white, navy, Great Northern), 1/2 cup seaweed, 1 tablespoon blackstrap molasses, 5 or more figs. *We recommend having 4-6 servings of healthy non-dairy sources of calcium rich foods daily.*

BEANS & LEGUMES: Are healthy protein foods. Vegetable protein foods are more optimal compared to animal protein foods (plant-based protein chart, see page 59). Vegetable proteins do not contain artery clogging saturated fats and cholesterol found in animal foods. They also contain protective factors to prevent heart disease, cancer and diabetes. Vegetable proteins provide the body with essential amino acids that it requires. One serving of vegetable protein foods include: 1 cup cooked legumes (beans, lentils, dried peas), 1/2 cup firm tofu or tempeh, 1 serving of "veggie meat" alternative veggieburger patty, 3 Tbsps. nut or seed butter, 1 cup soy, almond or rice milk. *We recommend 2-3 or more vegetable protein servings daily.*

53

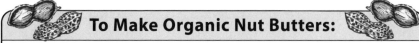

To Make Organic Nut Butters:

Grind 1 1/2 cups of raw unsalted organic nuts in a food processor or blender. Continue grinding nuts down until they are a thick, fudge-like paste. Then add sunflower or nut oil (start with 1 Tbsp. and add more only if necessary), blend until smooth. Best kept refrigerated.

Life cannot be maintained unless life is taken in. This is best done by making at least 60% of your diet raw and with a plentiful supply of fresh juicy organic fruits with some lightly cooked vegetables.
– Patricia Bragg

ESSENTIAL NUTRIENTS: are essential and healthy fats, like Omega-3's, vitamin D3 and minerals. Servings of healthy fats include: 1 tsp. of flaxseed oil, 1 Tbsp. of organic extra virgin olive oil, 3 tsps. of raw walnuts or pumpkin seeds. Other healthy essential nutrients include: ground flaxseeds or chia seeds and nutritional B-Complex supplements that provide vitamin B12. Do provide your body with nutritional supplements your body requires for optimal health and longevity!

What Are Nature's Miracle Phytonutrients?

These wonderful, organic compounds are found in plants, ('phyto' means 'plant' in Greek), that are vital to human health. Increasingly, Scientific Studies are showing that phytonutrients help protect us from many serious health issues, including heart disease and stroke. Organic fruits, vegetables, grains, legumes, nuts, seeds and some teas are rich in miracle phytonutrients.

54

Physicians and Scientists have written about the critical nature of these foods for thousands of years, but the specific benefits of phytonutrients are still being discovered. They are created when plants absorb energy from the earth, water, air and sun. This energy helps plants survive environmental challenges such as diseases, injuries, drought, excessive heat, ultraviolet sun rays and poisons. This incredible energy forms an important part of the plant's immune system! It appears to provide humans with the same benefits, when we consume the plants! They help increase our immune and regeneration systems. They give us strength, endurance, health and ultimately help us feel better and live longer.

WORLD'S HEALTHIEST FOODS RICH IN OMEGA-3 FATS

FOOD	% Daily Value	FOOD	% Daily Value
Flaxseeds	133%	Brussels Sprouts	11%
Walnut	113%	Winter Squash	8%
Chia Seeds	102%	Broccoli	8%
Soybeans	43%	Spinach	7%

CHIA SEEDS: Bragg promoted in 1940 – are rich in omega-3 fatty acids and antioxidants! Chia seeds provide fiber, calcium, phosphorus, magnesium, iron, niacin and zinc. They help slow down how fast our bodies convert carbohydrates into simple sugars, which may have benefits for diabetics.

Health Benefits of Phytonutrients

The body must have these phytonutrients and enzymes to break food down, kill viruses and bacteria and dissolve tumors! A diet of at least 50% raw, unprocessed foods is vital to make sure that we are getting enough enzymes and phytonutrients to optimize the body's processes.

Plants contain more than 10,000 phytonutrients, one reason 10-14 servings of organic fruits and veggies daily are vital! Plants and vegetables contain different phytonutrients, having a variety in your diet is important.

On average, plant foods have 64 times more antioxidants than animal foods, which is critical because when it comes to antioxidants, the more we eat, the more health benefits. Eating a diet high in antioxidants is important – they reduce inflammation in the body, they reduce free radicals and help protect against heart disease and cancer. See the chart on page 56 for health benefits of plant sources.

Main Sources of Miracle Phytonutrients

The following are high in phytonutrients: carrots and yellow vegetables (sweet potatoes, pumpkins, etc.), broccoli, red cabbage, leafy greens (kale, spinach, turnip greens), tomatoes, grapefruit, peaches, apricots, watermelon, guava, blackberries, strawberries, cranberries, raspberries, blueberries, grape juice, and prunes, pineapple, oranges, plums, kiwi fruit, red peppers, pinto beans and walnuts.

The more live, unprocessed foods we eat the more phytonutrients and enzymes we consume the healthier our diet. This natural food is full of energy we need to live longer, healthier lives! To boost your immune system and cell regeneration of the body, eat more phytonutrients, practice deep breathing exercises daily, get physical exercise, and make sure that your diet is at least 50% raw, healthy, organic foods. **That's The Bragg Healthy Lifestyle and when followed produces miracles.**

Increasing intake of fruits and vegetables can help prevent heart disease, cancer and other chronic diseases. Surveys show those who increase their daily fruit and vegetable intake improve their health, vitality and well-being.
– UC Berkeley Wellness Letter • www.BerkeleyWellness.com

Mother Nature's Miracle Phytonutrients Help Prevent Cancer

Make sure to get your daily dose of naturally occurring, cancer-fighting super foods – Phytonutrients are abundant in apples, tomatoes, onions, garlic, beans, legumes, soybeans, cabbage, cauliflower, broccoli, citrus, etc. Champions with highest count of Phytonutrients – apples and tomatoes.

Phytonutrient	Food Sources	Health Action
PHYTOESTROGEN ISOFLAVONES	Soy products, flaxseed, seeds and nuts, yams, alfalfa, pomegranates lentils, carrots, apples	Helps block some cancers, aids in menopausal symptoms, balances hormones, helps improve memory, enhances heart health
PHYTOSTEROLS	Plant oils: corn, sesame, safflower; rice bran, wheat germ, peanuts	Blocks hormonal role in cancers, inhibits uptake of cholesterol from diet, reduce risk of heart attack
LIGNANS	Flaxseeds, rye, lentils, soy mushrooms, barley	Helps prevent breast cancer, heart disease and balances hormones
SAPONINS	Yams, beets, beans, cabbage, nuts, soybeans	Helps prevent cancer cells from multiplying, reduces cholesterol
TERPENES	Carrots, winter squash, sweet potatoes, yams, apples, cantaloupes, cherries	Antioxidants – protects DNA from free radical-induced damage, and improves immunity
	Tomatoes and its sauces, tomato-based products	Helps block UVA & UVB and offers help to protect against cancers – breast, prostate, etc.
	Spinach, kale, beet and turnip greens, cabbage	Protects eyes from macular degeneration,
	Red chile peppers	Keeps carcinogens from binding to DNA
QUERCETIN (& FLAVONOIDS)	Apples (especially the skins), red onions and green tea	Strong cancer fighter, protects heart - arteries. Reduces pain, allergy and asthma symptoms
	Citrus fruits (flavonoids)	Promotes protective enzymes
PHENOLS	Apples, fennel, parsley, carrots, alfalfa, cabbage	Helps prevent blood clotting & has important anticancer properties
	Cinnamon	Promotes healthy blood sugar and glucose metabolism
	Citrus fruits, broccoli, cabbage, cucumbers, green peppers, tomatoes	Antioxidants – flavonoids, block membrane receptor sites for certain hormones
	Apples, grape seeds	Strong antioxidants; fights germs and bacteria, strengthens immune system, veins and capillaries
	Grapes, especially skins	Antioxidant, antimutagen; promotes detoxification. Acts as carcinogen inhibitors
	Yellow and green squash	Antihepatotoxic, antitumor
SULFUR COMPOUNDS	Onions and garlic, (fresh is always best) Red onions (our favorite) also contain Quercetin Onions help keep doctor away	Promotes liver enzymes, inhibits cholesterol synthesis, reduces triglycerides, lowers blood pressure improves immune response, fights infections, germs and parasites

Apples Are Powerful Phytonutrient Foods

"An apple a day keeps the doctor away," *a wise saying known to millions.* This carries truth and common sense, because apples are one of God's great health-giving foods and some say, *"Apples keep cancer away"* (chart page 56).

Apples are a rich source of potassium, as vital to soft tissues of the body as calcium is to bones and harder tissues. Potassium, the mineral of youthfulness is the "artery softener," keeping the body's arteries flexible and resilient. It fights viruses and bacteria. The apple has stood the test of time. It is one of the oldest known fruits that humans consume.

Eliminating Meat is Safer and Healthier

Play it safe, become a healthy vegetarian! We know that millions of people around the world eat meat. We also know that one out of every two deaths are caused by heart disease, heart attack and high blood pressure.

We never try to make our health students and readers vegetarians. The choice must be yours! We believe that by properly combining the natural foods, people can, if they strongly desire it, eat meat 1 - 2 times a week and still live a long, healthy life. Try to get only meats that are healthy and hormone-free and drug-free, etc. But we believe that the daily, heavy meat eaters can get into serious health and heart trouble! Fact: vegetarians live healthier and longer! Please keep the basic principles of The Bragg Healthy Lifestyle in mind at all times and keep adding more raw fruits and vegetables to your diet. Remember, fruits and vegetables are the great purifiers and the detoxifiers. Also **buy organic when possible – it's best in nutrition! Ask your green grocer to buy and stock organic produce!**

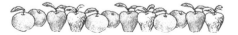

Eating apples gives you a burst of energy. Researchers found a significant boost in endurance capacity from quercetin in red apples. Quercetin (opposite page) is a natural antioxidant that boosts power of mitochondria (powerhouse of the cell) in muscles and the brain. This surge of power gives you energy!

"Now What About Protein?" You May Ask

If you feel you must eat meat, do so. Just remember, on this diet you don't eat meat more than 1-2 times a week. You can always have delicious vegetable proteins such as tofu, brown rice, beans, lentils, raw nuts and seeds (see next page). If you have bad teeth, raw nuts might be better ground or taken in the form of nut butters (recipe page 53) – same with raw seeds like sunflower, pumpkin, flax and sesame (*delicious sprinkled over salads, veggies, soups*). Buy a coffee grinder to grind raw nuts and seeds, and add flax or chia seeds for extra Omega 3s (see page 54).

Traces of protein are found in all foods (see next page). Just think, mother's milk is 3.5% protein and a new human body is built with this small amount of protein. We never worry about getting our daily quota of protein. The body is a miracle chemical factory and can easily convert other foods into protein. We don't believe in heavy animal protein diets! For over 50 years we've heard doctors and nutritionists declare the value of high-protein diets. But in our health work, we've found that many who did high-protein diets got into serious trouble (high blood pressures, heart trouble and strokes, gout, kidney, prostate and liver disorders).

To aid in the digestion of protein – drink 1 Tbsp. of organic apple cider vinegar (with the "mother" enzyme) in an 8 oz. glass of water, 15 minutes before eating, or take a digestive enzyme containing hydrochloric acid (HCL) with your meals. Many people do not make enough HCL in the stomach to fully digest protein, which causes gas, bloating, fatigue and blood sugar imbalances. Digestive enzymes are key to protein digestion.

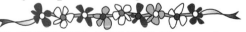

RACEHORSES ARE VEGETARIAN WINNERS! The racehorse does not eat concentrated protein. They get their great speed, strength and endurance from the vegetable kingdom. You can also eat raw nuts, seeds, raw wheat germ, beans, natural brown rices and lentils which are all wonderfully protein rich, healthy non-cholesterol and non-uric acid protein sources.

You must have protein for building every cell of your body. This basic function of your body – of converting food into living tissue – is one of life's miracles.

Plant-Based Protein Chart

BEANS & LEGUMES

(1 cup cooked)	PROTEIN IN GRAMS
Soybeans	29
Lentils	18
Adzuki Beans.	17
Cannellini	17
Navy Beans	16
Split Peas	16
Black Beans	15
Garbanzos (chick peas) . .	15
Kidney Beans.	15
Great Northern Beans . . .	15
Lima Beans	15
Black-eyed Peas	14
Pinto Beans	14
Mung Beans.	14
Tofu (3 oz.)	7 to 12
Green Peas (whole)	9

RAW NUTS & SEEDS

(1/4 cup or 4 Tbsps)	PROTEIN IN GRAMS
Chia Seeds.	12
Macadamia Nuts	11
Flax Seeds	8
Sunflower Seeds.	8
Almonds	7
Pumpkin Seeds	7
Sesame Seeds.	7
Walnuts.	5
Brazil Nuts.	5
Hazelnuts	5
Pine Nuts.	4
Cashews.	4

NUT BUTTERS

(2 Tbsps)	PROTEIN IN GRAMS
Peanut Butter	7 to 9
Almond Butter	5 to 8
Cashew Butter.	4 to 5
Sesame - Tahini	6

VEGETABLES

(1 Serving or 1 cup)	PROTEIN IN GRAMS
Spirulina	8.6
Corn (1 cob)	5
Potato (with skin)	5
Mushrooms, Oyster.	5
Artichoke (1 medium). . . .	4
Collard Greens	4
Broccoli	4
Brussel Sprouts	4
Mushrooms, Shiitake . . .	3.5
Swiss Chard.	3
Kale	2.5
Asparagus (5 spears)	2
String Beans.	2
Beets	2
Peas	2
Sweet Potato	3
Summer Squash.	2
Cabbage.	2
Carrot	2
Cauliflower	2
Squash	2
Celery	1
Spinach	1
Bell Peppers.	1
Cucumber	1
Eggplant	1
Leeks	1
Lettuce.	1
Tomato (1 medium)	1
Radish	1
Turnips	1

FRUITS

(1 Serving or 1 cup)	PROTEIN IN GRAMS
Avocado (1 medium).	4
Banana (1).	1 to 2
Blackberries (1 cup).	2
Pomegranate (1)	1.5
Blueberries (1 cup)	1
Cantaloupe (1 cup)	1
Cherries (1 cup).	1
Grapes (1 cup).	1
Honeydew (1 cup).	1
Kiwi (1 large)	1
Lemon (1)	1
Mango (1)	1
Nectarine (1)	1
Orange (1).	1
Peach (1)	1
Pear (1)	1
Pineapple (1 cup)	1
Plum (1).	1
Raspberries (1 cup)	1
Strawberries (1 cup).	1
Watermelon (1 cup)	1

GRAINS & RICE

(1 cup cooked)	PROTEIN IN GRAMS
Triticale	25
Millet.	8.4
Amaranth	7
Oat Bran	7
Wild Rice.	7
Couscous (whole wheat). .	6
Bulgur Wheat	6
Buckwheat.	6
Teff.	6
Oat Groats	6
Barley.	5
Quinoa	5
Brown Rice	5
Spelt.	5

DAIRY & NUT MILKS

(1 cup)	PROTEIN IN GRAMS
Soy Milk	6 to 9
Almond Milk.	1 to 2
Rice Milk	1
Eggs (1) *(free-range)*	6

59

This chart displays protein content of common vegetarian foods. Note that in order to determine amount of protein that is optimal for your body, use the following formula that is based on a vegan diet: *RDA recommends that we take in 0.36 grams of protein per pound that we weigh* (100 lbs. x 0.36 = 36 grams).

Data from webs: *TheHolyKale.com • VegParadise.com • vrg.org (Vegetarian Resource Group).*

Many vegetables, grains and legumes are excellent protein sources (chart previous page), including soybeans, tofu, brown and wild rice, lima beans, garbanzos, split peas, lentils, pinto and kidney beans. All beans are good sources of protein and magnesium and are important for a healthy heart and also wise "health insurance!"

If you desire meat, *(be sure it's hormone-free and drug-free)* limit it to 1 to 2 times weekly. Meat has uric acid, urea, saturated fats and cholesterol. These are toxic materials and not good for the heart and body. Fish *(be sure it is mercury free)* and free range poultry are cleaner proteins, with less saturated fat, uric acid and urea than red meat. Free-range poultry is better for you than red meat. **We prefer and urge you to learn to enjoy a heart-healthy vegetarian diet.**

Eggs *(free-range, fertile eggs are best)* if desired, limit to about 4 a week. If your count is over 200, leave eggs out until cholesterol gets to 180 or lower (see page 100). Milk cheeses are highly concentrated. If you eat cheese have naturally aged and feta (goat/sheep cheese) occasionally and forget processed cheese. Dairy products are mucus producing – eat them sparingly or not at all! Enjoy healthy soy cheeses instead.

Slowly cut down if you eat a heavy, unhealthy "meat" breakfast. Start eating fresh fruit, bananas, stewed prunes with raw wheat germ and soy yogurt for healthier breakfasts. Soon you can learn to eat lightly or not at all, for most people don't need breakfast. There weren't two people any more physically and mentally active than my father and me. We never ate breakfast, other than fresh fruit or our Bragg Healthy Energy Smoothie page 71. Upon arising we'd have our ACV drink (page 71). Before we ate we'd enjoy morning exercises, practicing our deep breathing or taking a hike or swim. Our day started early and we were busy until 9-10 am, before having our fruit or Energy Drink. Many mornings, we were so busy writing books for you, our readers, that we didn't even take time to eat! We've loved being Health Crusaders and sharing our Health Teachings with you!

Modern GMO Wheat – No Longer Mother Nature's Wheat!!!

Modern GMO wheat isn't really the wheat that Mother Nature intended. About 700 million tons of wheat are grown worldwide making it the second most-produced grain after corn. It's grown on more land area than any other commercial crop and considered a staple food for humans.

The Wheat We Eat Today Isn't the Wheat Our Grandmothers Ate!

The balance and ratio of nutrients "Mother Nature" has created for wheat has been modified! At some point in our history, this ancient grain was nutritious, however modern GMO wheat really isn't the same wheat at all. Once agribusiness took over to develop a higher-yielding crop, wheat became hybridized to the extent it has completely transformed from its prehistorical genetic configuration.

The majority of wheat is processed into 60% extraction or bleached white flour. The standard for most wheat products means that 40% of the original wheat grain is removed! So not only do we have an unhealthier, modified, and hybridized strain of wheat, we also remove and further degrade its nutritional value by processing it!

Unfortunately, the 40% that gets removed includes the bran and germ of the wheat grain – its most nutrient-rich parts. In the process of making 60% extraction flour, most of the vitamin B1, B2, B3, E, folic acid, calcium, phosphorus, zinc, copper, iron, and fiber sadly are lost. Any processed foods with GMO wheat are unhealthy since they cause more body health risks than benefits.

Heavily marketed white carbohydrates (white sugar, flour, pastas, etc.) that are packaged in boxes are designed to make you crave more. They're not good for the health of your body, mind or soul!

Seek out, and choose healthy whole foods: organic fruits, vegetables, rice, beans, nuts, seeds, etc. rather than the commercial, refined white flour and sugar products and highly processed canned goods in the center aisles.

People who turn away from GMO wheat have dropped substantial weight. People with arthritis have dramatic relief; and less acid reflux; leg swelling; and irritable bowel syndrome.

"The whiter the bread, the sooner you're dead!"

The body doesn't recognize processed GMO wheat as food. Nutrient absorption from processed wheat products is thus consequential with almost no nutritional value. Even if you choose 100% whole wheat products they are based on modern GMO wheat strains created by irradiation of wheat seeds and embryos with chemicals, gamma rays, and high-dose X-rays to induce mutations. You're still consuming genetically modified grain. To avoid all the toxic GMO wheat-oriented products, eat healthy foods – organic nuts, fruits and vegetables along with products made with non-GMO organic grains, or avoid wheat entirely if you discover it causes digestive distress.

Health Problems Associated With GMO Wheat

Dr. Marcia Alvarez who specializes in nutritional programs for obese patients says, "Modern GMO wheat grains could certainly be considered as the root of all evil in the World of Nutrition since they cause so many documented health problems across so many populations in the world." See web: *NonGMOproject.org*

Dr. Alvarez asserted that modern GMO wheat is now responsible for more intolerances than almost any other food in the world! "In my practice of over two decades, we have documented that for every ten people with digestive problems, obesity, irritable bowel syndrome, diabetes, arthritis and even heart disease, 8 out of 10 people have health problems with wheat! Once we remove modern GMO wheat from their diets, most of their symptoms disappear within 3 to 6 months," she added. Dr. Alvarez estimates that between the coming influx of genetically modified (GMO) strains of wheat and current growing tendency of wheat elimination worldwide, a trend is emerging in the next 20 years that will likely see 80% of people stop their consumption of GMO wheat in any form!

Fiber is vital for good health, healthy elimination and adequate intake helps prevent colon cancer! Everyone will benefit from making sure they regularly include foods in their diet such as organic non-GMO whole grains, barley, oats, beans, fruits and vegetables that provide healthy fiber.

Enjoy Healthy Fiber for Super Health

These are our suggestions for healthy fiber:

❯ EAT ALL VARIETIES OF ORGANIC BERRIES, surprisingly good sources of fiber.

❯ KEEP BEANS HANDY, probably the best fiber sources. Cook dried beans and freeze in portions. Use canned beans for faster meals.

❯ INSTEAD OF ICEBERG LETTUCE, choose deep green lettuces such as romaine, bib, butter, spinach or cabbage.

❯ LOOK FOR "100% ORGANIC WHOLE WHEAT" or whole grain breads, when eating bread.

❯ LOOK FOR WHOLE GRAIN or RICE CEREALS.

❯ GO FOR BROWN RICE over white rice.

❯ EAT THE SKIN of the potato, fruits and vegetables.

❯ SERVE HUMMUS, made from chickpeas, instead of sour-cream with your dip.

❯ DON'T UNDERESTIMATE NON-GMO ORGANIC CORN, especially popcorn and corn tortillas.

❯ ADD ORGANIC OAT BRAN & WHEAT-GERM to baked goods.

❯ SNACK ON ORGANIC SUN-DRIED FRUIT.

❯ INSTEAD OF DRINKING FRUIT JUICE, eat whole fruit.

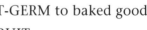

WARNING! Avoid All Unhealthy Microwaved Foods!

Microwaves deplete the nutrients in foods and can cause serious health issues. In the past 35 years (health destroying) microwaves have practically replaced traditional methods of cooking, especially with on-the-go people of today's world. But how much do we really know about them? A Swiss Study found that food which is microwaved is not the food it was before! Microwave radiation deforms and destroys the molecular structure of food – creating radiolytic compounds! Microwaves ruin as much as 60-90% of the energy in foods, including vitamins B12 and C. When microwaved food is eaten, abnormal changes occur in the blood and immune systems. These include a decrease in hemoglobin and white blood cell counts (which cause anemia) and an increase in cholesterol levels. Microwaving human milk damages the anti-infective properties it gives to babies. Microwaves can cause cataracts and digestive, liver, kidney, nervous system and brain damage. Many studies show increased cancer cells in blood and organs. Microwaving releases toxic chemicals from plastic or Styrofoam.
We never use microwaves. BEWARE: don't use microwaves!!

Watch Out for Hidden Sugars in Food Products

Food labelers often hide sugars in their products by calling them by other names. They also use more than one kind of sugar, so that sugar will not have to be listed first, as the most common ingredient. In a list of ingredients, sugar can often be called: corn syrup, corn sweetener, high fructose corn syrup, dextrose, fructose, glucose, sorbitol, mannitol, barley malt, grape sweetener, sorghum, lactose and maltose. If even two of these "hidden" sugars are listed as the third and fourth ingredients, it may be that sugar is actually the greatest ingredient in the product. *("The Healthy Heart Handbook" – Dr. Neal Pinckney)*

Beware of Toxic, Deadly Aspartame and Chemical Sugar Substitutes!

Although its name sounds "tame," this deadly Neurotoxin is anything but! Aspartame is an artificial sweetener (over 200 times sweeter than sugar) made by Monsanto Corporation and marketed as "Nutrasweet," "Equal," "Spoonful," and countless other trade names. Although Aspartame is added to over 9,000 food products, it's not fit for human consumption! This toxic poison changes into formaldehyde in the body and has been linked to migraines, seizures, vision loss and symptoms relating to Lupus, Parkinson's Disease, Multiple Sclerosis and other health destroying conditions! Besides being a deadly poison, Aspartame actually contributes to weight gain by causing a craving for carbohydrates. A study of 80,000 women by American Cancer Society found those who used this toxic "diet" sweetener actually gained more weight than those who didn't use Aspartame products.

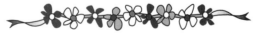

SUGAR IS SLOW SUICIDE: High sugar consumption can overstimulate and harm your whole body system. Research Studies revealed one of biggest hidden threats to health is consumption of fructose, sucrose, and all other forms of sugar, which can lead to many serious health problems, ranging from: obesity, cancer, and heart trouble, to high blood sugar levels and diabetes.– Dr. David Williams, "Guide to Healthy Living"

The Bragg Healthy Lifestyle helps make a Healthier You and a Healthier World.

High Fructose Corn Syrup (HFCS), is a highly toxic processed sugar, that contains similar amounts of unbound fructose and glucose. What makes HFCS unhealthy is that it's metabolized to fat in your body far more rapidly than any other sugar! It's a primary factor behind a number of health epidemics, including obesity, diabetes and heart disease. For a better sugar substitute use Stevia.

White Sugar Destroys Teeth, Bones & Health

The American fast food, junk food diet, in addition to lacking vitamins and minerals, is also highly acid-producing, due to the high proportions of refined white sugar, white flour and animal proteins, which increase acidity of the body with adverse effects on bones and health. Strong bones require an alkaline balance in body metabolism, naturally maintained by a higher proportion of raw organic fruits and vegetables in the diet. The worst villain is refined white sugar and its many products; there is no single food more devastating to the spine and other bones of the body. Sugar leaches calcium, phosphorus, magnesium and manganese out of the bones, making them weak, porous and brittle! Candy, sweets, refined white sugar products and all sugared drinks are prime causes of tooth decay and diabetes. Since teeth are the body's hardest tissue, you can understand what refined white sugar does to other bones and cartilages (protective cushions between bones) of the skeletal system, including the spinal column.

65

Stevia, A Safe Alternative to Sugar

Stevia – the natural herbal sweetener is an herb native to South America. It is widely grown for its sweet leaves. In its unprocessed form it is 30 times sweeter than sugar. It is a low carbohydrate, low-sugar food alternative. Stevia shows promise for treating such conditions as obesity and high blood pressure. It does not effect blood sugar and it even enhances glucose tolerance. It helps mental alertness, combats fatigue and improves digestion. Stevia is calorie-free and a safe, delicious, health sweetener for diabetics. Children can use Stevia without concerns, as it does not cause cavities.

For more information see website: *www.stevia.com*

The secret of longevity is eating intelligently. – Gaylord Hauser

Remember, LIVE FOODS produce healthy, LIVE PEOPLE!

Natural Healthy Foods Prevent Osteoporosis

When we were doing nutritional research along the Adriatic Coast of Italy, we found *ageless* men and women, advanced in calendar years, but whose bodies were youthful, supple and whose bones were firm, strong and resilient. Their diet consisted primarily of organic fresh salads, fresh fruits, raw and cooked vegetables, pastas, dark breads, olive oil, and natural cheeses rich in calcium, vitamins and minerals, all essential for strong bones! In our extensive research on nutrition, we rarely found osteoporosis among active people who lived on a simple diet of live, natural healthy foods.

Milk is Not a Good Source of Calcium

Nearly everyone has the idea that the problem of calcium deficiency will be solved if they just drink milk. This is not completely true. In the first place, practically all milk in U.S. is pasteurized, which robs and greatly reduces the availability of milk's calcium. (see web: *NotMilk.com*)

Dr. Harold D. Lynch – famous author, researcher and physician – said recently, *"Almost fanatic use of milk as a beverage has added more complications than benefits to child nutrition."* He further states, *"Milk may often be a primary cause of poor nutrition in children!"*

Most All Natural Foods Are Rich in Calcium

There are many fine sources of calcium other than milk (page 53)! We prefer the calcium found in kale, spinach, corn, beans, veggies, soy tofu and sesame seeds. In fact, as Dr. Lynch and Dr. Neal Barnard point out, all natural foods contain appreciable amounts of important calcium.

Read 2 important books on milk and why best to avoid:

- *Mad Cows and Milk* Gate by Virgil Hulse, M.D.
- *Milk, the Deadly Poison* by Robert Cohen

Also visit these websites:
- *www.NotMilk.com*
- *pcrm.org* (Physicians Committee for Responsible Medicine)

The first requisite of a good life is to be a healthy person. – Herbert Spencer

Locations in the Body Where Osteoporosis, Arthritis, Pain and Misery Hit the Hardest

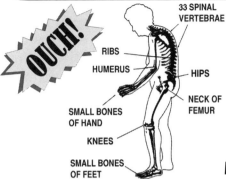

33 SPINAL VERTEBRAE

RIBS

HUMERUS

HIPS

NECK OF FEMUR

SMALL BONES OF HAND

KNEES

SMALL BONES OF FEET

OUCH!

OSTEOPOROSIS
Affects over 60 Million and Kills 400,000 Americans Annually Estimated 50% of adults 65 years or older also suffer from Arthritis.

Boron: Miracle Trace Mineral For Healthy Bones

BORON – An important trace mineral for healthier and stronger bones that also helps the body absorb more vital calcium, minerals and necessary hormones! Good Boron sources are most organic veggies, fresh and sun-dried fruits, avocados, prunes, raw nuts and soybeans.

The U.S. Dept. of Agriculture's Nutrition Lab in Grand Forks, ND, says Boron is usually found in soil and foods, but many Americans eat a diet low in Boron. They conducted a 17 week study which showed a daily 3 to 6 mgs. Boron supplement enabled participants to reduce loss (demineralization) of calcium, phosphorus and magnesium from their bodies. This loss is usually caused by eating processed fast foods, drinking tap waters (distilled is best), eating lots of meat, salt, sugar and fat and a dietary lack of fresh vegetables, fruits and whole grains. (*all-natural.com*)

Scientific studies show women benefit from a healthy lifestyle that includes vitamin D3 sunshine and exercise (even weight-lifting) to maintain healthier bones, combined with distilled water, low-fat, high-fiber, carbohydrates, and fresh organic fruits, salads, sprouts, greens and vegetable diet. This lifestyle helps protect against heart disease, high blood pressure, cancer and many other ailments! I'm happy to see science now agrees with my father who first stated these health truths in the 1920's.

For more hormone and osteoporosis facts, read pioneer, Dr. John R. Lee's book – "What Your Doctor May Not Tell You About Menopause"

Boron helps keep the skeletal structure strong by adding to bone density, preventing Osteoporosis, treating Arthritis and improving strength and muscle mass. Boron helps facilitate calcium directly into the bones. Boron protects bones by regulating Estrogen function. Boron is naturally found in beans, nuts, avocados, berries, plums, oranges and grapes. Boron helps relieve menopause symptoms and PMS. – Dr. Axe

It's Proven – Light Eaters Live Longer

My father's research and interviews with people who remained vigorous at ages over 100 years revealed that they ate sparingly, never over-ate and chewed thoroughly! Their diets were well-balanced with simple, natural foods. Scientific tests made on controlled animal feeding have also proven that light eaters live longer and in better health.

Always give thanks first, (millions are starving), then chew food slowly and thoroughly (your stomach has no teeth)! **Never eat in a hurry!** Food bolted down overworks the stomach, intestines and heart! If you don't have time to eat correctly, skip that meal! Fasting (pages 129-139), shows skipping a meal is a good habit to develop when needed.

Large Waist-Lines Lead to Shorter Life-Spans

Surplus weight in the belly lessens physical activity and often mental activity, too. Don't be satisfied thinking that a naturally fatty surplus comes with advancing years! Beware if you make this mistake, then old age arrives sooner coupled with serious illness and premature death.

> *Overeating puts more strain on the heart than any other one thing! Many people load up on a ten-course dinner and soon afterward suffer a heart attack! Overeating is a dangerous, deadly habit that can lead to serious consequences! You should make it a habit to always get up from the table feeling that you could eat a little more!*

If you're sporting a large waistline, risk of dying prematurely is nearly double! Reason is because belly fat, often referred to as "spare tire" sends out toxic streams of chemicals impacting the whole body. Waist size over 35" in women and over 40" in men greatly increases risk of chronic diseases like diabetes, heart disease and more. – DoctorOz.com

Research shows that Concord grapes, blueberries, fruits and veggies in a rainbow of colors are rich in polypheno! compounds that help reduce heart disease, cancer, asthma, Alzheimer's.

They also help to keep your blood vessels and arteries flexible and healthy, including your brain which enhances memory!

Food and Product Summary

Today, many of our foods are highly processed or refined, robbing them of essential nutrients, vitamins, minerals and enzymes. Many also contain harmful, toxic and dangerous chemicals. Research findings and experience of top Nutritionists, Physicians and Dentists have led to the discovery that devitalized foods are a major cause of poor health, illness, cancer and premature death! The enormous increase in the last 70 years of degenerative diseases such as heart disease, arthritis, diabetes and dental decay, backs this belief. Scientific Research shows most of these afflictions can be prevented and others, once established, can be arrested or even reversed through nutritional methods.

Enjoy Super Health with Natural Foods

1. **RAW FOODS:** Fresh fruits and raw vegetables organically grown are always best! Enjoy nutritious variety garden salads with raw vegetables, sprouts, raw nuts and seeds.

2. **VEGETABLES and PROTEINS:**
   a. Legumes, lentils, brown rice, soy beans, and all beans.
   b. Nuts and seeds, raw and unsalted (lightly roasted okay).
   c. We prefer healthier vegetarian proteins. If you must have animal protein, then be sure it's hormone–free, and organically fed and no more than 1 or 2 times a week.
   d. Dairy products – fertile range-free eggs (*4 weekly*), unprocessed hard cheese and feta goat's cheese. We choose not to use dairy products. Try the healthier non-dairy soy, rice, coconut, and almond milks and soy cheeses, delicious soy yogurt and soy and rice ice cream.

3. **FRUITS and VEGETABLES:** Organically grown is always best – grown without the use of poisonous sprays and toxic chemical fertilizers whenever possible; do urge your markets to stock healthier organic produce! Steam, bake, sauté and wok vegetables as short a time as possible to retain the best nutritional content and flavor. Also enjoy fresh juices.

4. **ORGANIC non-GMO WHOLE GRAINS, CEREALS, BREADS:** Barley, rye, buckwheat, spelt, teff, oatmeal, quinoa, millet, amaranth, wild rice, etc. contain important B-complex vitamins, vitamin E, minerals, fiber and unsaturated fatty acids.

5. **COLD or EXPELLER-PRESSED VEGETABLE OILS:** Organic, first press, extra virgin olive oil (is best), soy, flax, sunflower, and sesame oils are good sources of healthy, essential, unsaturated fatty acids. We still use oils sparingly.

Feed Your Pets as Well as You Do Yourself!

A man at 70 really might have only lived half his lifetime! We support this statement with the fact that most animals live from 5-7 times their rate of maturity. Years ago we had an older pet dog that was about to go into heat. Determined that she would bear the healthiest litter possible, we fed her an extra super-balanced nutritional diet, supplemented with vitamins. We kept one of her pups and called him "Vitamin." He was a healthy and beautiful pup. We kept him that way throughout his many years of life by feeding him only nutritious foods.

Our buddy and friend "Vitamin" enjoyed eating almost everything we ate: beans, brown rice, lentils, carrots and other vegetables – these we mixed with his healthily-prepared dog food. We also sprinkled over his food good quality Nutritional Yeast Flakes (nutritious in B-complex vitamins, boron, etc.) to enhance his health and it helped keep fleas away. He liked his water "spiked" with a dash of organic raw apple cider vinegar which helped keep his body germ-free! ACV also helped keep his body limber and free from the stiffness of arthritis.

Most dogs and cats enjoy small slices of raw beef heart and chewing on large bones, and so did "Vitamin." To this day all our dogs and cats live a very healthy life.

Here's "Angel," my faithful friend for almost two decades. We kept her in good health on the same program "Vitamin" followed. Daily she was brushed, massaged and exercised. She loved fast walking and running, and was never sick, fat or mean. Her teeth were perfect and her breath was sweet. She pranced, ran and wagged her tail when she was excited, like a puppy. Angel knew she was loved and appreciated!

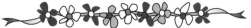

Flea collars and shampoos contain pesticides that are toxic to pets and humans. Instead use a soft leather collar and essential oils such as citronella, rosemary and rose geranium to repel fleas and ticks. This is only for dogs, sorry cats can't tolerate essential oils. Use for dogs only!

Angel

HEALTHY BEVERAGES
Fresh Juices, Herb Teas & Energy Drinks

These freshly squeezed organic vegetable and fruit juices are important to *The Bragg Healthy Lifestyle*. It's not wise to drink beverages with your main meals, as it dilutes the digestive juices. But it's great during the day to have a glass of freshly squeezed orange juice, grapefruit juice, vegetable juice, raw, organic apple cider vinegar drink (see below), or herbal tea – these are all ideal pick-me-up beverages.

Apple Cider Vinegar Drink – Mix 1-2 tsps. raw, organic apple cider vinegar (with the 'Mother' enzyme) and (optional) to taste raw honey or pure maple syrup *(if diabetic, to sweeten use 2 stevia drops)* in 8 oz. of distilled or purified water. Take glass upon arising, an hour before lunch and dinner.

Delicious Hot or Cold Cider Drink – Add 2-3 cinnamon sticks and 4 cloves to water and boil. Steep 20 minutes or more. Before serving add raw organic apple cider vinegar and sweetener to taste.

Bragg's Favorite Juice Drink – This drink consists of all raw vegetables *(remember organic is best)* which we prepare in our juicer / blender: carrots, celery, cucumber, beets, cabbage, tomatoes, watercress, kale, parsley, or any vegetable combination you prefer. The great purifier, garlic we enjoy, but it's optional.

Bragg's Favorite Healthy Energy Smoothie – After our morning stretch and exercises we often enjoy the drink below instead of fruit. It's a delicious and powerfully nutritious meal anytime: lunch, dinner or in a thermos at work, school, sports, the gym and during sports or hikes. You can freeze for popsicles too.

Bragg's Favorite Healthy Energy Smoothie

Prepare the following in a blender, add frozen juice cubes if desired colder; Choice of: freshly squeezed orange or grapefruit juice; carrot and greens juice; unsweetened pineapple juice; or $1^1/2$ - 2 cups purified or distilled water with:

2 tsps spirulina or green powder
$1/3$ tsp Nutritional Yeast
2 dates or prunes-pitted
1 tsp protein powder (optional)

1-2 bananas or fresh fruit
1-2 tsps almond or nut butter
1 tsp flaxseed oil or grind seeds
1 tsp raw honey (optional)

Optional: 4-6 apricots (sun-dried,) soak in jar overnight in purified water or unsweetened pineapple juice. We soak enough to last for several days. Keep refrigerated. In summer you can add organic fresh fruit: peaches, papaya, blueberries, strawberries, all berries, apricots, etc. instead of banana. In winter, add apples, kiwi, oranges, tangelos, persimmons or pears, and if fresh is unavailable, try sugar-free, frozen organic fruits. Serves 1 to 2.

Patricia's Delicious Health Popcorn

Use freshly popped organic popcorn (use air popper). Drizzle organic olive oil, melted coconut oil or salt-free butter over popcorn. Sprinkle with good quality nutritional yeast for amazing flavor. For a variety try a pinch of cayenne pepper, mustard powder or fresh crushed garlic to oil mixture. Serve instead of breads!

Healthy, healing dietary fibers are organic fresh vegetables, fruits, salads whole grains and their products. These health builders help normalize your blood pressure, cholesterol and promotes healthy elimination

Lentil & Brown Rice Casserole, Burgers or Soup
Paul Bragg and Jack LaLanne's Favorite Recipe

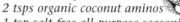

16 oz pkg organic lentils, uncooked   4 garlic cloves, chop
1 cup brown organic rice, uncooked   2 onions, chop
5 cups, distilled / purified water   2 tsps organic coconut aminos
4-6 carrots, chop $^1/_2$" rounds   1 tsp salt-free all-purpose seasoning
3 celery stalks, chop   2 tsps organic extra-virgin olive oil
1 cup diced fresh or canned tomatoes (salt-free)

Wash and drain lentils and rice. Place grains in large stainless steel pot. Add water, bring to boil, reduce heat and simmer 30 minutes. Now add vegetables and seasonings and cook on low heat until tender. Last five minutes add fresh or canned (salt-free) tomatoes. For delicious garnish, add minced parsley. **For Burgers mash. For Soup, add more water in cooking grains.** Serves 4 to 6.

Raw Organic Vegetable Health Salad

2 stalks celery, chop $^1/_2$ cup red cabbage, chop
1 bell pepper & seeds, dice $^1/_2$ cup alfalfa, mung or sunflower sprouts
$^1/_2$ cucumber, slice   2 spring onions & green tops, chop
2 carrots, grate   1 turnip, grate
1 raw beet, grate   1 avocado (ripe)
1 cup green cabbage, chop   3 tomatoes, medium size

For variety add organic raw zucchini, peas, mushrooms, broccoli, cauliflower, (try black olives and pasta). Chop, slice or grate vegetables fine to medium for variety in size. Mix vegetables & serve on bed of lettuce, spinach, chopped kale or cabbage. Dice avocado and tomato and serve on side as a dressing. Serve choice of fresh squeezed lemon, orange or dressing separately. Chill salad plates before serving. **It's best to always eat salad first before hot dishes.** Serves 3 to 5.

72

Patricia's Health Salad Dressing

$^1/_2$ cup raw organic apple cider vinegar $^1/_2$ tsp organic coconut aminos
1-2 tsps organic raw honey   1-2 cloves garlic, minced
$^1/_3$ cup organic extra-virgin olive oil, or blend with safflower, soy, sesame or flax oil
1 Tbsp fresh herbs, minced (to taste)

Blend ingredients in blender or jar. Refrigerate in covered jar.

For delicious Herbal Vinegar: In quart jar add $^1/_3$ cup tightly packed, crushed fresh sweet basil, tarragon, dill, oregano, or any fresh herbs desired, combined or singly (If dried herbs, use 1-2 tsps herbs). Now cover to top with raw, organic apple cider vinegar and store two weeks in warm place, and then strain and refrigerate.

Honey – Chia or Celery Seed Vinaigrette

$^1/_4$ tsp dry mustard   1 cup organic apple cider vinegar
$^1/_4$ tsp organic coconut aminos $^1/_2$ cup organic extra-virgin olive oil
$^1/_4$ tsp paprika or to taste $^1/_2$ small onion, minced
1-2 Tbsps honey $^1/_3$ tsp chia or celery seed (or vary to taste)

Blend ingredients in blender or jar. Refrigerate in covered jar.

Studies show both beta carotene and vitamin C, abundantly found in fruits and vegetables, play vital roles in preventing heart disease and cancers.

Allergies & Dr. Coca's Pulse Test

Almost every known food may cause some allergic reaction at times. Thus, foods used in *elimination* diets may cause allergic reactions in some individuals. Some are listed among the *Most Common Food Allergies* (see below). Since reaction to these foods is generally low, they are widely used in making test diets. By keeping a food journal and tracking your pulse rate after meals you will soon know your *problem* foods. Allergic foods cause pulse to then go up. (Take base pulse, for 1 minute, before meals, then 30 minutes after meals, and also before bed. If it increases 8-10 beats per minute – check foods for allergies.)

If your body has a reaction after eating some particular food, especially if it happens each time you eat that food, you may have an allergy. Some allergic reactions are: wheezing, sneezing, stuffy nose, nasal drip or mucus, dark circles, eye watering or bags under your eyes, headaches, feeling light-headed or dizzy, fast heart beat, stomach or chest pains, diarrhea, extreme thirst, breaking out in a rash, swelling of extremities or stomach bloating. **Do read Dr. Arthur Coca's book, *The Pulse Test.***

If you know what you're allergic to, you are lucky; if you don't, you had better find out as fast as possible and eliminate all irritating foods from your diet. To re-evaluate your daily life and have a health guide to your future, start a daily journal (keep a notebook – enlarge and copy form on next page) of foods eaten, your pulse rate before and after meals and your reactions, moods, energy levels, weight, elimination and sleep patterns. You will discover the foods and situations causing problems. **By charting your diet you will be amazed at the effects of eating certain foods. We have kept daily journals for years.**

If you are hypersensitive to certain foods, you must omit them from your diet! There are hundreds of allergies and of course it's impossible here to take up each one. Many have allergies to milk, wheat, or some are allergic to all grains. **Visit web: *FoodAllergy.org*. Your daily journal will help you discover and accurately pinpoint the foods and situations causing you problems. Start your journal today!**

Most Common Food Allergies

- **DAIRY:** Butter, Cheese, Cottage Cheese, Ice Cream, Milk, Yogurt, etc.
- **CEREALS & GRAINS:** Wheat, Corn, Buckwheat, Oats, Rye
- **EGGS:** Cakes, Custards, Dressings, Mayonnaise, Noodles
- **FISH:** Shellfish, Crabs, Lobster, Shrimp, Shad Roe
- **MEATS:** Bacon, Beef, Chicken, Pork, Sausage, Veal, Smoked Products
- **FRUITS:** Citrus Fruits, Melons, Strawberries
- **NUTS:** Peanuts, Pecans, Walnuts, chemically dried preserved nuts
- **MISCELLANEOUS:** Chocolate, Cocoa, Coffee, Black & Green (caffeine) Teas, Palm & Cottonseed Oils, MSG & Salt.

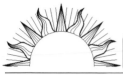

MY DAILY HEALTH JOURNAL

Today is:____/____/____

> *I have said my morning resolve and am ready to practice faithfully The Bragg Healthy Lifestyle today and every day.*

Yesterday I went to bed at: Today I arose at: Weight:

Today I practiced the No-Heavy Breakfast or No-Breakfast Plan: ☐ yes ☐ no

- For Breakfast I drank: Time:

  For Breakfast I ate:
                                          Time:

  Supplements:

- For Lunch I ate: Time:

  Supplements:

- For Dinner I ate: Time:

  Supplements:

- ____ Glasses of Water I Drank during the Day, including ACV Drinks

  List Snacks – Type and When:

  _____

- I took part in these physical activities (walking, gym, etc.) today:

  _____

Grade each on scale of 1 to 10 (desired optimum health is 10).

- I rate my day for the following categories:

Previous Night's Sleep:	Stress/Anxiety:
Energy Level:	Elimination:
Physical Activity, Exercise:	Health:
Peacefulness:	Accomplishments:
Happiness:	Self-Esteem:

- General Comments, Reactions and any To-Do List:

Chapter 6

You Must Breathe Deeply of Mother Nature's Pure Air!

When You Breathe Deeply and More Fully You Live Healthier, Happier, Longer Lives

When you pump a generous flow of oxygen into your body, 100 trillion cells become more alive! This enables the four main *motors* of your body – the heart, lungs, liver and kidneys – to operate and perform better. Your miracle-working bloodstream purifies and cleanses every part of the body, including itself. This eliminates toxic wastes as Mother Nature planned, and the fuel (food) and vital oxygen are carried to every cell in your body.

With ample oxygen your muscles, tendons and joints function more smoothly! Your skin becomes firmer and more resilient and your complexion clearer and more glowing. You will then radiate with greater health and well-being for a longer, healthier life!

With the *Bragg Super Power Breathing* your brain becomes more alert and your nervous system functions better. You become free from tension and strain because you can easily take the stresses and pressures of daily living. Your emotions come under control. You feel joyous and exuberant. If negative emotions such as anger, hate, jealousy, greed or fear intrude, you can expel them by positive thinking and slow, concentrated deep breathing.

The deep breather enjoys more peace of mind and body, tranquility and serenity. In India, the great teachers practice deep, full breathing as the first essential step towards higher spiritual development! You can attain higher concentration in prayers and meditation by taking long, slow, deep breaths. Also, deep breathing stimulates your brain cells and promotes new brain cell growth.

Breathing deeply, fully and completely energizes the body, calms the nerves, fills you with peace and helps keep you healthier and more youthful.
– Paul C. Bragg, N.D., Ph.D., Life Extension Pioneer

Super Deep Breathing Improves Brain Power

One of the main solutions to creating more energy and better body and brain functioning lies in healthy foods and with living a healthy lifestyle. Deep breathing constantly cleanses and purifies the body. Unobstructed oxygen circulation and maintaining a vital, healthy elasticity of the cells and tissues is vitally important. The person who breathes deeply and fully thinks more clearly and sharply! Oxygen stimulates your brain and logic and intelligence! The more deeply and fully you breathe, the greater your power of concentration and the more your creative mind asserts itself. You will also develop greater extrasensory perception within your body, especially the brain. Scientists at the Salk Institute for Biological Studies, in La Jolla, California, now know adults do generate new brain cells in the hippocampus, an area in the brain which is responsible for learning and memory. Deep breathing nourishes and fine-tunes the brain and the entire body! (*salk.edu*)

76

With a clean, purified body and an ample supply of oxygen you can enjoy a more youthful, energetic healthful body for a longer life. Read Bragg's book *Super Power Breathing*. The more fully and deeply you breathe, the further you will travel to higher levels on the physical, mental and spiritual planes. Now close your eyes. Relax and take a few minutes while doing some slow, deep breathing!

Directions for Filling the Entire Lungs With Life-Giving Oxygen

Lie flat on your back, either in bed or on the floor, relax and then slowly inhale through your nose and do not consciously try to move the upper chest or the abdominal region. While you are inhaling, place your hands on your lower ribs, which are known as the floating ribs. Now – if you are breathing correctly – you can feel your lower ribs expand. Slowly take in a long, deep breath. When you feel that your lungs are filled to full capacity with air – then you can slowly expel the breath with a long, lip-pursed sigh. Pause for 10 seconds, then repeat routine. Do 15 breathing exercises in the morning and at night. Visit web: *www.doctoroz.com* for more relaxing breathing techniques.

Deep Breathers Live Longer & Healthier

Air is one of the most important energizers of the human body. The more deeply you breathe pure air, the better your chances are for extending your life on this earth. For over 75 years, we have done extensive research on long-lived people and discovered the one common denominator among them all – they are deep breathers! We have found that the deeper, therefore fewer breaths a person takes in one minute, the longer they live.

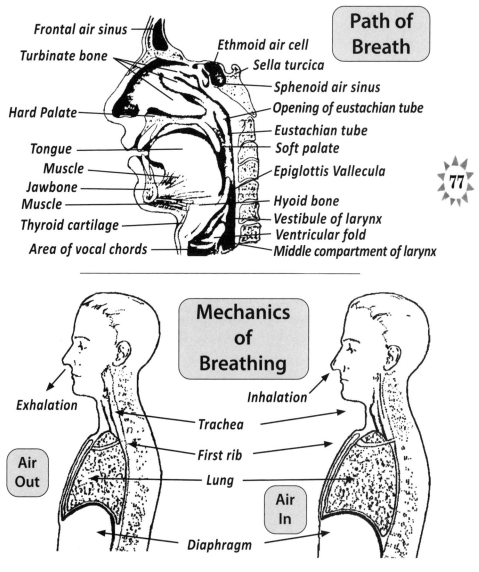

Path of Breath

Frontal air sinus
Turbinate bone
Hard Palate
Tongue
Muscle
Jawbone
Muscle
Thyroid cartilage
Area of vocal chords

Ethmoid air cell
Sella turcica
Sphenoid air sinus
Opening of eustachian tube
Eustachian tube
Soft palate
Epiglottis Vallecula
Hyoid bone
Vestibule of larynx
Ventricular fold
Middle compartment of larynx

77

Mechanics of Breathing

Exhalation
Air Out

Inhalation
Air In

Trachea
First rib
Lung
Diaphragm

Mechanics of Breathing, showing diaphragm position and flexible ribs at exhalation and at inhalation.

Super Power Breathing Promotes a Healthy Body

The most important of all physical acts is proper breathing. The rhythm and depth of breath directly affects the state of your mind and body health. You can not be 100% healthy if you do not breathe deeply. Taking deeper breaths will bring more oxygen into your body and improve your energy levels! Deep breathing is not only important for living longer, but also towards having a happy life and to keep performing at your best.

Here are health benefits of deep breathing and why you should make it a part of your daily living:

★ *Deep Breathing Detoxifies and Releases Toxins.* The body is designed to release 70% of its toxins through breathing. If you are not breathing effectively, you are not ridding your body of toxins! The more toxic poison you burn up, the more vitality you will create!

★ *All Internal Organs are Massaged.* The movements of the diaphragm during deep breathing exercise massages the stomach, small intestine, liver and the pancreas.

★ *Respiratory System Works Better.* Respiratory diseases like asthma, bronchitis, Chronic Obstructive Pulmonary Disease, emphysema and even chest pain can subside.

★ *Digestive System Does Its Job.* Digestive ills (poor digestion, bloating, constipation) are helped by the internal massage of correct diaphragmatic action. When Super Power Breath is taken, the digestive tract gets healthy exercise. Deep optimal breathing is the great body health normalizer. Oxygen, the invisible staff of life, is food for the body and helps with assimilation of foods! Oxygen burns calories and helps promote normal, healthy weight. The digestive organs receive more oxygen, and hence then operate more efficiently.

STOP CHEWING GUM – It Causes Stomach and Digestive Problems: Please never chew gum – it fools the body into thinking food is coming. Gum chewing starts digestive juices flowing. These powerful juices can cause trouble with your empty stomach's lining, resulting in stomach ulcer problems, IBS, heartburn, bloating, gas, etc. The habit of chewing gum may also increase your junk-food intake, trigger TMJ in your jaw, cause tooth decay (even sugar-free gum), and may release mercury from your fillings.

★ *Lymph System Works Better.* Increases circulation of lymphatic fluid which speeds recovery after illnesses.

★ *Circulation System Moves!* Many people suffer from poor circulation in various parts of the body. Because they don't get sufficient oxygen to produce steady blood circulation into their extremities, they have cold hands, feet, noses and ears. **The more oxygen you get into your body, the better it is for your circulation, heart, and your hands and feet will be warmer!** When more oxygen gets into your bloodstream, you will feel super energized and have greater vitality to better enjoy a longer, healthier, happier life! See web: *breathing.com*

★ *Immune System has More Energy.* **Deep Breathing creates more energy for the body to heal and detoxify.** Helps tissues to regenerate and heal. Enriches your blood cells to metabolize nutrients and vitamins. Super Power Breathing is now a part of all cures. Today, in the modern hospital, pure oxygen can heal many conditions when every other method of healing has failed. Even broken bones heal more quickly when the blood is purified by doing daily Super Power Breathing Exercises. Oxygen – the great invisible food for life, stimulant and purifier – builds our health resistance to infections and strengthens our weak points. It's our most vital aid in helping the body to heal itself and to stay healthy!

★ *Cleansing Systems Work Better.* Excess fluids are eliminated through deep breathing. The stress on organs is lessened, allowing the body to cleanse naturally.

★ *Blood Quality Improves.* When you breathe in oxygen correctly, you add millions of health-giving, oxygen-carrying red blood cells to your bloodstream, your miracle river of life. Deep Breathing removes all the carbon-dioxide and increases oxygen in the blood.

★ *Nervous System Improves.* The brain, spinal cord and nerves receive increased oxygen. This improves the health of the whole body, since the nervous system communicates to all parts of the body. Many nervous diseases are due to oxygen starvation. Deep, diaphragmatic breathing tranquilizes jangled nerves, stimulates the brain with clear thinking and more alertness to help solve many of life's problems and to help you make wise decisions.

★ *Lungs are Strengthened.* When you fill your lungs with more miracle-working oxygen, you cleanse your body of toxic poisons that could do your body great health damage. As you breathe deeply, lungs become healthier and more powerful. Good insurance against respiratory problems.

★ *Heart Grows Stronger.* Slow, deep breaths soothe and recharge the heart. Conversely, rapid, shallow breathing exhausts it through overwork and lack of sufficient oxygen for the blood. Since the heart doesn't have to work as hard to deliver oxygen to the tissues, the heart can rest a little.

★ *Muscles Get a Workout.* When you breathe easier you move easier! Deep breathing increases flexibility and strengthens joints and supplies oxygen to the brain and all cells in your body which increases the growth of the muscles in your body.

★ *Emotionally You Feel Better.* People who deeply inhale larger amounts of oxygen are happier people. Super Power Breathing cleanses your body of psychological and physical poisons and provides more joyful daily living and emotional well-being.

80

★ *Reduces Feelings of Stress.* Deep breathing relaxes the body and releases endorphins – natural pain-killers that create natural highs – and makes it easier to sleep. Deep breathing will help clear uneasy feelings out of your body.

★ *You Become Mentally Present.* Mental observation and concentration is improved. There is greater productivity, insight and learning and better decision making.

★ *Physical Appearance Improves.* People who get ample oxygen sleep better and have better muscle tone. Skin is healthier, firmer and more alive! Oxygen is Mother Nature's great miracle beautifier. It gives the skin a radiant glow and the hair a lustrous sheen.

You will have fewer wrinkles from improved circulation. Breathing helps create beautiful skin at any age! Good breathing techniques will also encourage good posture, which in turn helps you to look and feel younger (see posture exercise page 89). If you are overweight, the extra oxygen helps burn up excess fat more efficiently.

Breathing is the greatest pleasure in life. – Papini, 1881-1956

Life is in the breath. He who half breathes, half lives! – Old Proverb

★ *Increases Your Spirituality.* Deep Breathing deepens your meditation and increases your intuition when you're relaxed. Helps connect you to your inner soul which helps with "self-love" and greater compassion for others.

★ *Promotes Super Energy!* You will no longer crave artificial stimulants (caffeine, alcohol, tobacco) when sufficient oxygen is taken into your system. Oxygen is the wise stimulant that has no harmful after-effects.

The Importance of Clean Air to Health

It's essential to breathe pure, clean air – air that is as free as possible from such chemicals as smog, car exhaust, natural gas appliance fumes, off-gassing fumes, and the many other toxic chemical pollutants. Also, our air needs to be as free as possible from mold, dust, dust mites and their fecal matter, animal dander and pollen! Everyone's health is helped in varying degrees by clean air. **It's vitally important to live and work in an area which has clean air and is free of all harmful fumes.** It's also equally important to keep our homes pure, clean and free from dust, dust mites and debris! **Most people cannot be truly 100% healthy until they breathe clean air, maintain a healthy diet and live a healthy lifestyle.**

81

Live Longer Breathing Clean Air Deeply

We advise those who live and work in smog-ridden, polluted cities to obtain a good air filter. We especially recommend filters which contain charcoal and a high efficiency particulate HEPA air filter. The charcoal removes most of the chemicals and the HEPA filter removes most of the particles. To be effective in an average room, the flow rate through the filter should be over 200 cubic feet of air per minute. The wise motorist will also install an air filter in his car for cleaning the air while driving in air-polluted cities. These can be found at auto part stores or online.

"Being optimistic is like a muscle that gets stronger with use. It makes it easier when tough times arrive. You have to change the way you think in order to change the way you feel." – Robin Roberts, author, "Everybody's Got Something" and anchor on ABC's morning show – "Good Morning America"

When we are born, our lungs are new, fresh, clean, and rosy in color. If we could live in a dust-free atmosphere breathing deeply all our lives, then our lungs would remain *as good as new* for a long, healthy lifetime of use. Yet most people abuse their lungs! Some of this comes from external causes. The miracle lungs are the only organs of the body which are directly affected by external conditions, specifically, by the air we breathe into them!

Mother Nature has provided protection against a normal amount of dust contamination: tiny hairs in the nose serve as filters and moist mucus in the passages leading to the lungs trap dust particles that we expel through the nose or mouth. The lungs protect themselves remarkably well by expelling carbon dioxide through oxygenation and by discharging toxins into the blood for elimination via the kidneys. ***Your body is a miracle!***

Unfortunately, most civilized people today live in very unnatural conditions! Almost everywhere there are abnormal amounts of pollutants in the air we breathe, especially in city areas. Our lungs are often overloaded with more contaminants than they can handle! These are passed along into the bloodstream and to other body parts. The lungs of modern city dwellers become brownish from car smog, soot, smoke, etc. Even in most farming areas, the lungs must contend with pollens, excessive dust, poisonous pesticides, fertilizers and other toxic chemicals.

Deadly Smoking – A Health Hazard to Avoid – What it Does to You and Those Around You!

When people inhale deadly tobacco smoke into their miracle lungs, the protective cilia hairs filter out much of the smoke's harmful substances before it is exhaled. This means that while harmful toxins are trapped in the delicate linings of the smokers' lungs, fewer of these toxins are re-released into the air for others to breathe in. However, between a smoker's deadly puffs, the cigarette burns directly into the air. This smoke is known as "secondhand" or "side-stream" smoke, but it should be called "direct" smoke. Smoke that burns directly into the air is completely unfiltered and more deadly than the smokers' smoke! Stay away from all deadly smoke!

Recent studies establish that people who live or work around smokers are more likely to develop lung and sinus damage than smokers! For asthma or bronchitis sufferers, this exposure is very damaging. In addition to these dangers, "direct" smoke irritates eyes, nose and throat and smells up everything it comes in contact with (rooms, hotels, offices, carpets, drapes, cars and everything around smoking).

For the cigarette smoker, whose miracle lungs have unfortunately become the filters protecting the body from the deadly smoke, the effects are equally – if not more – damaging. Tar begins to collect in the lungs once there is too much to be removed through the lungs' normal cleaning processes. This means the over-burdened lungs can no longer clean normal contaminants they have to deal with. Dirt inhaled into the alveoli – which is normally trapped in a layer of sticky mucus and carried out of the lungs by the wavelike motions of the tiny cilia hairs – becomes trapped and stuck in the lungs. The cilia hairs become paralyzed by tar, so the normal cleansing (drain) procedures break down and the airways become clogged. This makes the lungs resort to coughing, spitting and respiratory – breathing attacks, flu, etc. in an effort to expel the contaminated, clogging toxins, tar and mucus.

There is good news! When a person stops smoking the cilia hairs begin to heal and move again. Smokers – stop now, you begin cleansing and healing immediately!

SMOKING HAS MANY WAYS TO KILL YOU!

The body has no defense against carbon monoxide produced by smoking. The coal tars in tobacco are the chief poisons responsible for cancer of the lungs, mouth and related areas of the body. It frightens us to think of what will happen in another 25 years because of excessive use of tobacco. We are convinced that every smoker (cigar also) will develop lung, throat esophagus or some other form of cancer, if heart disease doesn't kill them first.

If you smoke and already have heart disease, quitting will reduce your risk of dying from heart disease. Over time, quitting will also lower your risk of atherosclerosis and blood clots. FACT: According to the CDC, lung cancer is responsible for 28% of smoking related deaths while 43% are attributable to cardiovascular disease and strokes!

Please visit websites: • www.cdc.gov/tobacco • BeTobaccoFree.hhs.gov • lung.org for more info on smoking and damage it does to your lungs!

Quit Smoking – See the Difference it Makes!

- **20 MINUTES AFTER QUITTING:** Your blood pressure, heart rate and pulse rate drop to normal levels. The temperature of your hands and feet increases to normal.

- **8 HOURS AFTER QUITTING:** Carbon monoxide (which can be toxic to your body) decreases to lower levels and your blood oxygen levels increase to normal.

- **24 HOURS AFTER QUITTING:** You substantially lessen your chances of having a heart attack or stroke.

- **48 HOURS AFTER QUITTING:** Your nerve endings start regrowing and your ability to taste and smell is enhanced.

- **2 WEEKS TO 3 MONTHS AFTER QUITTING:** Nicotine will now be out of your body. Your circulation improves. Brisk walking, physical activity and exercise becomes easier. Your lung function increases as much as 30%.

- **1 TO 9 MONTHS AFTER QUITTING:** You will be able to exercise and perform physical activities without feeling winded and sick. Coughing, sinus congestion, fatigue and shortness of breath decreases. Your lungs and body are becoming cleaner and more resistant to infection.

- **1 YEAR AFTER QUITTING:** You will no longer have withdrawal symptoms. Excess risk for coronary heart disease decreases to an amazing 50% that of a smoker's.

- **2 TO 3 YEARS AFTER QUITTING:** Risk for heart disease and stroke decrease compared to those of people who have never smoked. Also less chance of osteoporosis.

- **5 YEARS AFTER QUITTING:** Lung cancer death rate for former one-pack-a-day smoker decreases by almost half. Risk of having a stroke reduces, risk of developing mouth and throat cancer is half that of a smoker.

- **10 TO 15 YEARS AFTER QUITTING:** Lung cancer death rate is almost that of non-smokers. Pre-cancerous cells are replaced. Risks for mouth, throat, esophagus, bladder, kidney, breast and pancreas cancer have decreased. Risk of developing diabetes is now similar to that of a person who has never smoked.

– Prevention Magazine • www.prevention.com

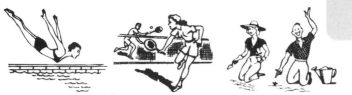

Chapter 7

You Must Exercise the 640 Muscles of Your Body

The Great Health Importance of Exercising

You have roughly 640 muscles and all these muscles must be used! If you do not use them, you lose them! If they are not used, they then start to lose their tone, strength and flexibility! There are hundreds of ways to exercise the human body. The best and greatest of all exercise is brisk walking – no special equipment is required except good walking shoes. You can walk vigorously, swinging your arms, for a good workout or just take a stroll. When you walk and breathe in deeply as you stride along you are building Vital Force and stimulating the eliminating and cleansing processes. After walking, swimming is the second-greatest exercise. Any sport that brings into play the muscles of the body can be part of your daily healthy lifestyle. Tennis and even gardening are considered wonderful exercise. You should also have a 20 to 30 minute daily exercise program of stretching, aerobics and super power breathing exercises (page 76).

Daily Exercise Helps Keep You Healthy

We are 100% for physical fitness and exercise! We think the ideal combination of natural nutrition, multi vitamin-mineral supplements (especially vitamin E) and exercise can work wonders for a person. We love hiking, swimming, tennis, mountain climbing, progressive weight-training and most forms of exercise, plus organic gardening! Every day of our lives we should look forward to some physical activity. To over-rest is to rust! If you don't use your muscles – your muscles will lose their firmness, tone and strength. But we also realize our bodies must be kept clean of toxic poisons by our weekly 24 hour detox water fast plus, 3 or 4 times a year, plan a fast lasting from 7 to 10 days.

When you follow The Bragg Healthy Lifestyle, you are filled with inexhaustible vitality and energy! You are like a child who is healthy and you become an active, healthy and happy person! You love life and activity: walking, swimming, biking, gardening, etc. and keep active regardless of your calendar years! You forget your calendar age and become ageless and tireless! – It's fun!!!

Big Muscles Don't Prove You're Healthy!

Just because men and women are athletic or powerfully built with great strength and endurance does not mean that they are internally clean! Far from it. Many athletic people overeat on the heavy, stimulating foods. We know weightlifters who eat 4 or 5 pounds of meat daily, drink quarts of milk and stuff other heavy, stimulating foods into their stomach. They feel it gives them big, powerful muscles and great physical powers. But we have also seen many of those former athletes die in their early 50s and 60s. No, not all athletes necessarily live longer than others! When they stop their heavy exercising – thus slowing down their circulation – the toxic poisons build up from their diet of heavy proteins, fats, refined sugars, etc. This causes an overall slowdown in their protein-burdened body. The toxic poisons are no longer being continually flushed out by the heavy exercising, which they stopped. As the toxins accumulate, they start to suffer from the same ailments that the non-athletic person endures!

Some think it's only strong muscle mass or physical fitness that counts. But it all comes down to the question: *"How Clean and Healthy is your body internally?"*

Self improvements have been shown to be effective to help you accept yourself for what you are and feel positive for what you see in yourself and your future goals! Goals practiced daily for about 15 minutes are more productive than spending all your waking hours fighting to lose weight, or other negatives you find in yourself. During self hypnosis (self-guidance) tell yourself to let go all the bad feelings about yourself, breathe deeply, then relax. Concentrate on feeling comfortable about each area of your body and tell yourself to treat yourself more lovingly. When you can forgive yourself, you'll be able to forgive others easier and feel better about yourself and everyone around you! This helps you become motivated into loving action to improve your entire lifestyle on all levels!

What Miracles Exercise Can Do for You

Get outdoors fast and get physically active when you feel dark moods, anxieties, worries, blues, depression and tensions overtaking you – otherwise these negative moods can damage you! Walking or any other outdoor exercise will help clear up your thinking and put your problems in perspective. Any form of outdoor recreation recreates the human personality. The ancient holy men of India believed the body and bloodstream had to be pure and strong before this could become a reality. Thus, they developed a physical fitness system called Yoga. They practice their belief daily, that the body is meant to be stretched, strengthened and exercised correctly in order to remain healthy. No matter what your calendar years, start turning back your biological clock now faithfully with exercise.

The Benefits of Being Fit and Healthy

The benefit of being fit and keeping active, is an improved quality of life – being able to do things you enjoy for longer periods of time. To be fit, one must have good habits! This includes eating healthy foods like organic fruits and vegetables, exercising regularly, getting enough sleep and being clean. Becoming fit will help you tremendously both physically and mentally. As you become more fit these benefits will happen:

Looking Better: weight loss, toned muscles, better posture.

Feeling Better: more energy, better sleep, better able to cope with stress, reduced depression and anxiety, increased mental sharpness, and fewer aches and pains.

Being Healthier: more efficient heart and lungs, lower cholesterol, lower blood pressure, ability to heal faster, stronger bones with less risk of osteoporosis, less stress on joints, better balance and flexibility, strengthened immune system, and reduced risk of dying early, heart disease, obesity, diabetes, cancers, and strokes. (*www.icb2001.com*)

Exercising just 15 minutes or more a day helps maintain healthy blood vessels for good circulation in the body and brain and helps you manage your weight and stress levels. Studies have shown that brisk walking helps delay brain shrinkage that delays the onset of dementia.

More Benefits of Daily Exercise:

1. **Exercise increases circulation**, and brings more oxygen into your body. You will feel more energetic.

2. **Exercise relieves stress**, strain and tension. Tension gets locked in the tight, stiffened areas of your body, especially the neck, back and spine. Exercise will stretch and loosen these areas as it restores youthful limberness. You will feel more relaxed and at ease.

3. **Overcoming chronic tiredness** is a major benefit of exercise. That chronic tired feeling to a great extent is due to a lack of sufficient circulation to your brain. Exercise brings the oxygen-laden blood into this vital area with an energizing and revitalizing effect.

4. **Exercise helps calm the nerves.** Nothing can calm the nerves better than 30 minutes of brisk walking and exercise. It also helps to promote a good night's sleep, which is absolutely essential to maintaining calmness, repose, serenity and health.

5. **Exercise increases emotional control.** Exercise helps to strengthen the nerves of the body and helps create healthy composure that comes from a healthy nervous system and a balanced, happy state of mind.

Exercise Promotes Health & Youthfulness

We know that healthy living with proper exercise can produce a new caliber of men and women who will enjoy more strength to carry out their daily work and have sufficient energy left for after-work interests, family and hobbies. They can retain the prime of life for 20 to 40 years longer than the person who does not exercise! Examples: both Tom Selleck and Clint Eastwood exercise, lift weights and eat healthy.

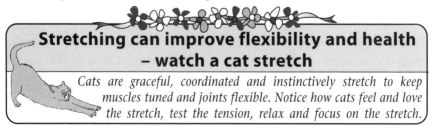

Stretching can improve flexibility and health – watch a cat stretch

Cats are graceful, coordinated and instinctively stretch to keep muscles tuned and joints flexible. Notice how cats feel and love the stretch, test the tension, relax and focus on the stretch.

Observe and respect your body and the Laws of Mother Nature.

All external characteristics of health (such as powerful Nerve Force) are but the result of the healthy functioning of your vital internal organs and glands. These are what keep you going. Exercise actually extends into your body bringing about miracle improvements in certain internal areas such as your nervous system, your heart, liver, lungs, kidneys, entire digestive tract, colon and thyroid gland among others. To attain these benefits you should faithfully follow a regular program of exercise.

Good Posture Important For Health & Looks

To maintain oneself in a healthy state involves many factors: the right natural food, rest, exercise, sleep, fasting, control of emotions and mind and, last but not least, good posture. If a body is properly nourished and cared for, good posture is not a problem. When the body lacks the essentials, poor posture is often the result. Once poor habits have been established, one must faithfully practice corrective exercises and good posture habits daily.

Bragg Posture Exercise Gives Instant Youthfulness

Tighten the butt, suck in the stomach muscles, lift up your ribcage and stretch up the spine. Keep the chest up and out, shoulders back and lift the chin up slightly and line the spine up straight (nose plumbline straight to belly button). Drop the hands to the sides and swing your arms to normalize your posture. Do this exercise before a mirror and see miraculous changes. You are retraining and strengthening your muscles to sit, stand and walk tall and straight for more youthfulness and health!

Good Posture – First Step to Healthy Living

Poor posture puts your heart, lungs and all of your *working machinery* into a viselike grip which impairs operations, circulation and efficiency. Keep saying to yourself, *"I must stretch up tall and lift up my chest and diaphragm."* Now, you will be exercising during all of your waking hours. Good posture brings inner strength and tone to your organs and muscles that no exercise can provide.

It's never too late to begin getting into shape, but it does take daily perseverance! – Dr. Thomas K. Cureton, Professor, University of Illinois, World Physical Fitness Expert, Researcher Fitness Council – 5 U.S. Presidents

WHERE DO YOU STAND?

POSTURE CHART

	PERFECT	FAIR	POOR
HEAD			
SHOULDERS			
SPINE			
HIPS			
ANKLES			
NECK			
UPPER BACK			
TRUNK			
ABDOMEN			
LOWER BACK			

90

Your posture carries you through life from your head to your feet. This is your human vehicle and you are truly a miracle! Cherish, respect and protect it by living The Bragg Healthy Lifestyle. – Patricia Bragg

Remember – Your posture can make or break your health!

Correct posture is vital for health and longevity! Keep a straight line from the chin to the toes when standing. Don't slump in your chair when sitting. Keep the head, chest and diaphragm held high. This may tire you at first, but only because your unused muscles are being re-awakened and trained! Once you give strength and tone to the many muscles that control your posture (some also help hold your internal organs), you will find it's easy to maintain good posture. The health rewards are many and you will look and feel healthier and more youthful.

The Dangers of Sitting Too Long

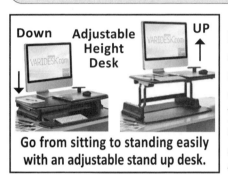

Go from sitting to standing easily with an adjustable stand up desk.

People who sit for too long at home or work may develop a thrombosis (blood clot) in the deep veins of the calf. If office work requires you to sit long hours at a computer, *get up, move around every half hour or get this desk.*

Don't Cross Your Legs – It's Unhealthy

When sitting – never cross your legs! Under the knees run two of the largest arteries, called popliteal arteries carrying nourishing blood to the muscles below the knees and to nerves in the feet. You immediately cut down the blood flow to a trickle when you cross your legs.

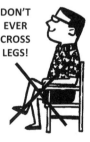

DON'T EVER CROSS LEGS!

When the muscles of the legs and knees are not nourished and don't have good circulation, then the extremities stagnate, which can lead to varicose veins or broken capillaries and other problems. People who are habitual leg-crossers have more acid crystals stored in the feet than those who never cross their legs. Crossing the legs is one of the worst postural habits of man. It throws the hips, spine and head off balance and it's the most common cause of chronic backaches, headaches and varicose veins. Be kind to your body – please don't cross your legs. You can break this habit.

Walk Off Your Emotional Tensions

We learned many years ago that we could actually walk off our emotional strains. No matter how serious the problems we faced, we could find the answer to our dilemma in a brisk 2-to 4-mile walk. Some of the greatest decisions we have had to make in our lives were made during one of our hikes. As the oxygen floods into the body from vigorous walking, one can think more clearly.

A wealthy friend telephoned Dad during the great financial depression of the 1930s and said, "Paul, I am completely ruined financially. I am going to kill myself, and I called up to say good-bye." My father asked this tormented man to grant him just one favor. When he agreed, Dad said, "All right, we will have a walk and a farewell talk before you end your life." Dad got in his car, dashed to his friend's home and off they went, hiking for a full five hours. During that time father told him that money was not the only thing in life and that he had to get some perspective and straighten out his values! Dad literally walked some sense into him! Had that man stayed at home and brooded over his loses, he would have destroyed himself, but that long nature walk in fresh air changed his whole life! Dad's friend was not rich materially, but rich in inner wealth.

Exercise is the Best Fitness Conditioner

A daily program of walking, running or jogging is a quick, sure and inexpensive fitness conditioner! Be faithful to your exercise routine for true heart fitness. Women will be especially pleased when they see fat change to firmness, as the inches fly off their waistlines and hip-lines – all the while improving their health! Men and women, please remember your waistline is your lifeline and also your dateline! A person with a trim and fit figure always looks more youthful and attractive!

A good laugh, a walk and a long sleep are the best cures in the doctor's book!

Exercise helps you lose and control weight in two ways. First, by elevating your metabolism you burn more calories. Second, by building muscle – which requires more energy to maintain – you use even more calories. Exercising promotes better elimination and circulation that helps body cleansing!

If you feel you cannot get outside for your run or jog on cold and rainy days – stationary indoor jogging to music or your favorite show will work too. Stay in one place and lift one foot at a time about 6-8 inches from floor – it's best to start easy and gradually build up to faster, longer periods. Remember to exercise where you get the most fresh air – on the patio, front porch, or inside or outside rest areas at work.

Enjoy Exercising – It's Healthy and Fun!

There is great hiking near where we had a home in Hollywood, California, where Mt. Hollywood rises some 1,600 feet in famous Griffith Park. We enjoyed early morning hikes up the mountain to greet the sun rising and would then run down. Also, in Santa Barbara, California, we always enjoy an ocean swim and hiking in the surrounding foothills.

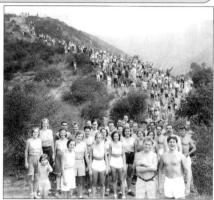

A thousand Happy Bragg Health Students enjoy hiking, exercise and fresh air on the trail to Mt. Hollywood, CA, summer, 1932.

We love to walk, jog and climb mountains. We make time to walk or jog daily, or we swim, play tennis or ride our bikes. We work out 3 times a week with a progressive weight training program, which helps keep our bones and muscles healthier and stronger. See pages 97-99.

Exercise is the greatest single health factor available to us that helps us remove any blockages and unclog the arteries and blood vessels, and for increasing the vital flow of oxygen-enriched blood throughout the heart and body! Recent studies show that exercise improves health and also reduces the risk of developing adult-onset diabetes as well as breast cancer. The Harvard School of Public Health Researchers (*www.health.harvard.edu*) studied 70,000 women. Results: 46% lowered their risk of diabetes with daily vigorous exercising and brisk walking.

The strongest principle of growth lies in the human choice. – George Elliot

Laughter is inner jogging, and good for your body and soul. – Norman Cousins

The Importance of Abdominal Exercises

We believe that the most important exercises are those that stimulate all of the muscles of the human trunk from the hips to the armpits. These are the binding muscles which hold all of the vital organs in place. When you develop your torso's muscles, you are also developing your internal muscles and posture. As your back, waist, chest and abdomen increase in strength and elasticity, so will your lungs, heart, stomach, kidneys, etc. gain in efficiency. Please be faithful with your exercising!

The widened arch of your ribs will give free play to your lungs. Your elastic diaphragm will allow your heart to pump more powerfully. Your rubber-like waist will, in its limber action, stimulate your kidneys and massage your liver. Your abdominal muscles will strengthen and support your stomach with controlled undulations. All of this strong, clean development of your torso will stimulate and help maintain the sound walls of your house and fortify the interior to resist the ravages of time. Trunk exercise acts like a massage of the vital organs, for that reason alone, it has a positive influence over the whole body that cannot be underestimated.

20 Year Study Shows Being Fit Saves Money

The average American spends over $9,600 on health care yearly, and costs are rising! (Forbes and CNBC) This revealing 20 year study done by Dr. Tedd Mitchell of Cooper Clinic monitored 6,679 men. Results showed those who exercised more, required fewer doctor visits. Being fit cuts yearly medical expenses 25 to 60%. The study also found all you need to stay fit is to exercise just 20 to 30 minutes a day, four or five days a week. Physically fit people live longer and enjoy a better quality of life!
Visit web: *CooperWellness.com*

Positive affirmations create miracles. – Beatrex Quntanna

Make fitness a lifestyle with Flex™ Heart Monitor – WIRELESS ACTIVITY and SLEEP WRISTBAND. This slim wristband device you wear as often as you want, keeps track of your walking distance and even calories burned. If worn at night, it tracks your sleep quality and wakes you silently in the morning. It's the motivation you need to get walking and be more active!
– Check out web: FitBit.com

Enjoy Exercise & Jogs for Happy, Long Life

On our around-the-world Bragg Health Crusades the first question we would ask the hotel manager was, where is the nearest park where we can take our daily exercise? And off we would go sometime during the day. We preferred to go early in the morning or late in the afternoon. Each person, however, should choose the time best suited and available to them.

We were so pleased to find that all over the world walking, hiking, running and jogging have become an accepted method in the pursuit of Heart Fitness by people of all age groups. Many cities have walking, hiking and jogging clubs. We have enjoyed running with folks world-wide; including Europe, England, Australia, New Zealand and throughout the USA.

It's universally accepted exercise benefits are important for physical, mental and emotional health. A daily run or jog when adapted to an individual's physical condition and age will improve endurance, produce a sense of well-being and help to maintain total body fitness (each step gives your trillions of cells a massage, also try trampolining and stationary jogging while watching TV). Exercise helps increase resistance to sickness and disease, and helps make the heart stronger and life longer!

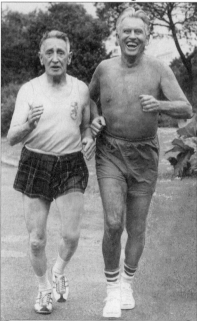

Before starting on your exercise program, it's wise to seek advice from your health practitioner. Also, be sure that you choose a soft surface to run or jog on, such as grass or sand. Jogging on hard surfaces, such as concrete and asphalt, add to an accumulation of repetitive damage to your knees, hips, ankles and other organs.

Bragg with friend Duncan McLean, England's oldest Champion Sprinter, (83 years young) on a training run in London's beautiful Regent's Park.

Duncan McLean & Paul C. Bragg

Is Age a Hindrance to Daily Exercise?

The answer is unequivocally, "No!" In fact, age is no excuse for not exercising! Our friend Roy White, 106 years young, walked 3-8 miles daily. No one is too old to continue safe exercise (see following study). Conrad Hilton jogged for years (see page 30).

To rest is to rust! It is far better to wear out than to rust out. The saying, *If you don't use it, you lose it,* certainly applies to the 640 muscles of the body. When you don't exercise regularly, your muscles lose their supple tone. As soon as you put down this book go outdoors and take a brisk, invigorating walk. Say out loud while walking: *Health! Peace! Joy! Love for Eternity!* You will feel great and your trillions of cells will rejoice with circulation!

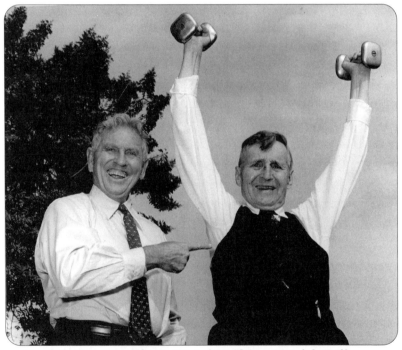

Paul C. Bragg and His Weight Lifting Health Follower
My father's good friend, Roy White of Long Beach, California, had a tireless, painless and ageless body. He knew the Laws of Mother Nature and he lived by them. He didn't fear old age. We both could name many more friends who are in their 80s, 90s and even over 100, who are biologically youthful!

 The best way to lengthen life is to avoid shortening it!
Start exercising and living a healthy lifestyle!

Iron-Pumping Oldsters (ages 86 to 96) Triple Their Muscle Strength In Landmark U.S. Government Study

WASHINGTON NEWS — Ageing nursing home residents in Boston *pumping iron?* Elderly weightlifters tripling and quadrupling their muscle strength? Is it possible? Most people would doubt and wonder at this amazing revelation!

Yet the government experts on ageing answered those questions with a resounding *"yes"* according to the results of this study. They turned a group of frail Boston nursing home residents, aged 86 to 96, into weight-lifters to demonstrate that it's never too late to reverse age-related declines in muscle strength. The study group participated in a regime of high-intensity weight-training research conducted by the Agriculture Departments Human Research Center of Ageing at Tufts University in Boston. *A high-intensity weight training program is capable of inducing dramatic increases in the muscle strength in frail men and women up to 96 years of age.* This was reported by Dr. Maria A. Fiatarone, the Study Director.

97

Amazing Health & Fitness Results in 8 Weeks

The favorable response to strength training in these subjects was remarkable in light of their very advanced age, extremely sedentary habits, many chronic diseases, functional disabilities and nutritional inadequacies.

Despite their many handicaps, the elderly weight lifters increased their muscle strength by 3 to 4 times in as little as 8 weeks. Dr. Fiatarone said they were stronger at the end of the program than they had been in years!

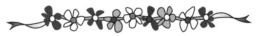

Studies show repeatedly that exercise – particularly impact exercises like brisk walking, tennis, square dancing, cycling, aerobics and weight lifting – help you maintain a healthier heart, body and build stronger bones!

The three greatest letters in the English alphabet are N-O-W. There is no time like the present. So begin Now!
– Sir Walter Scott, Explorer and Scottish Poet, 18th Century

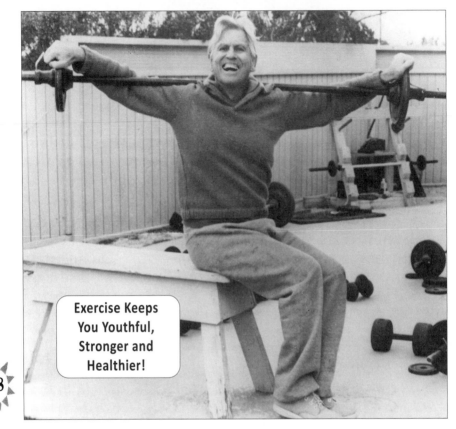

Exercise Keeps
You Youthful,
Stronger and
Healthier!

Paul C. Bragg and Patricia enjoyed lifting weights 3 times weekly.

Dr. Fiatarone and associates emphasized the safety of such a closely supervised weight lifting program, even among people in frail health. The average age of the ten participants was 90. Six had coronary heart disease, seven had arthritis, six had bone fractures resulting from osteoporosis, four had high blood pressure, and all had been physically inactive for years. Yet no serious medical problems resulted from this program. A few participants did report minor muscle and joint aches, but 9 of the 10 still completed the program.

The study participants, drawn from a 712-bed long-term care facility in Boston, worked out three times a week during the study. They performed three sets of eight repetitions with each leg on a weight lifting machine. The weights were gradually increased from 10 pounds to about 40 pounds at the end of the eight week program.

Exercise, along with healthy foods and some fasting helps maintain or restore a healthy physical balance and normal weight for a long, happy life.

Dr. Fiatarone said the study carries potentially important implications for older people, who represent a growing proportion of the population. A decline in muscle strength and size is one of the more predictable features of ageing! Muscle strength in the average adult decreases by 30% to 50% during the course of a lifetime. Experts on ageing do not know whether the decrease is an unavoidable consequence of ageing, or results mainly from a sedentary lifestyle and other controllable factors.

Macfadden – Founder of Physical Culture

My dad worked closely with Bernarr Macfadden and together they changed the entire health culture in America. While Dad was the father of the Health Movement and the originator of health food stores, Macfadden was known as the father of physical culture in America. He founded the *"Physical Culture Magazine,"* the first of its kind in the country. My father served as the editor of the magazine, which brought the basic principles of healthful living to popular attention in America. They were credited with "getting women out of bloomers into shorts, and men into bathing trunks." Macfadden started "Penny Kitchen Restaurants" during the big Depression Era, when they fed millions of hungry people for a penny each. Bragg helped Macfadden with his Miami Health Spa Hotel: The Macfadden – Deauville Hotel.

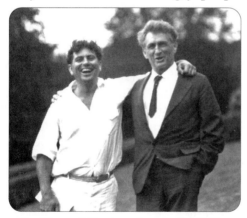

Paul Bragg & Mentor – Bernarr Macfadden

My dad was associated for many years with Macfadden, who spent thousands of dollars to find the oldest living humans on earth. Dad was his main researcher on this project. This took him to many very interesting, remote parts of the world, interviewing men and women from 103 to 120 years of age! Dad found this work fascinating, because he loved promoting health and longevity, that not just the life of the average person which ends at about 77, but an active life that would last 120 to 150 years (Genesis 6:3). The Bragg research proved it can be done! Now Scientists worldwide are agreeing.

Age does not depend upon years, but upon lifestyle and health!

HEALTHY HEART HABITS FOR LONG, VITAL LIFE

Remember, *organic live foods make live people. You are what you eat, drink, breathe, think, say and do.* So eat a low-fat, low-sugar, high-fiber diet of organic fresh raw salads, sprouts, greens, vegetables, whole grains, fruits, raw seeds, nuts, fresh juices and chemical-free, purified or distilled water.

Earn your food with daily exercise. For regular exercise, brisk walking, improves your health, stamina, go-power, flexibility, endurance and helps open the cardiovascular system! Only 45 minutes a day truly can do miracles for your heart, arteries, mind, nerves, soul and body! You become revitalized with new zest for living to accomplish your life goals!

We are made of tubes. To help keep them open, clean and to maintain good elimination, I take 1 veg psyllium cap or add 1 tsp psyllium husk powder daily an hour after dinner to juices, herbal teas, even apple cider vinegar drink. I also take one Cayenne capsule (40,000 HU) daily with a meal. I also take 50 to 100 mgs. regular-released Niacin (B3) with one meal daily to help cleanse and open the cardiovascular system; also improves memory. Skin flushing may occur, don't worry about this as it shows it's working! After cholesterol level reaches 180, then only take Niacin twice weekly.

The heart needs healthy balanced nutrients, so take natural multi-vitamin-mineral food supplements: Omega-3 and extra heart helpers – vitamin E with mixed tocotrienols; vitamin C; Ubiquinol CoQ10; vitamin D3; MSM; D-Ribose; garlic; turmeric; selenium; zinc; beta carotene and amino acids – L-Carnitine, L-Taurine, L-Lysine and Proline. Folic acid, CoQ10, vitamin B6 and B12 helps keep homocysteine level low. Magnesium orotate, hawthorn berry extract helps bring relief for palpitations, arrhythmia, senile hearts and coronary disease. Take multi-digestive enzyme and probiotics with meals; it aids in digestion, assimilation and elimination.

100

For sleep problems try 5-HTP tryptophan (an amino acid), melatonin, calcium, magnesium, valerian (in capsule, extract or tea), and Sleepytime herb tea. For arthritis or joint pain/stiffness, try aloe juice or gel, glucosamine-chondroitin-MSM combo caps and shots, helps heal and regenerate. Capsaicin and DMSO lotion helps relieve pain. Natural liver cleanses to repair and regenerate include: milk thistle; dandelion root; artichoke and turmeric. Dandelion root is a natural diuretic and helps clear toxins through urination and also helps stimulate liver bile flow so waste can be eliminated.

Use amazing antioxidants – E Tocotrienols, vitamin C, quercetin, grape seed extract (OPCs), CoQ10, selenium, SOD, resveratrol, and alpha-lipoic acid. They improve immune system and help flush out dangerous free radicals that cause havoc with cardiovascular pipes and health. Research shows antioxidants promote longevity, slow ageing, fight toxins, help prevent disease, cancer, cataracts and exhaustion.

Recommended Heart Health Tests (for Adults):

- **Total Cholesterol:** 180 mg/dl or less is optimal
- **LDL Cholesterol:** 130 mg/dl or less is optimal • **HDL Cholesterol:** 50 mg/dl or more
- **Triglycerides:** 150 mg/dl or less is normal level
- **HDL/Cholesterol Ratio:** 5.0 or less • **Triglycerides/HDL Ratio:** below 2
- **Homocysteine:** 6-9 micromoles/L
- **CRP (C-Reactive Protein high sensitivity):**
  - 1 mg/L = low risk • 1-3 mg/L = average risk • over 3 mg/L = high risk
- **Diabetic Risk Tests:**
  - **Glucose:** (do 12 hour food fast) 80-100 mg/dl • **Hemoglobin A1c:** 6% or less
- **Blood Pressure:** 120/70 mmHg is good for adults

Chapter 8

You Must Give Your Body Pure, Safe Clean Water

Pure Distilled Water Is Important for Health

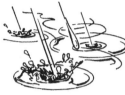

To the days of the aged it addeth length;
To the might of the strong it addeth strength;
It freshens the heart, it brings us delight;
It's like drinking a goblet of morning light.

The body is 75% water and purified or steam-distilled (chemical-free) water is important for total health. You should drink 8-9 glasses of water a day. Read our book *Water – The Shocking Truth* for more information on the importance of pure water.

Pure distilled water is vitally important in following The Bragg Healthy Lifestyle. Water is the key to all body functions including: digestion, circulation, bones and joints, assimilation, elimination, energy, muscles, heart, nerves, metabolism, glands and senses. The right kind of water is one of your best natural protections against all kinds of diseases and viral infections, such as influenza and pneumonia. It is a vital factor in all body fluids, tissues, cells, lymph, blood and all glandular secretions. Water holds all nutritive factors in solution, as well as toxins and body wastes, and acts as the main transportation medium throughout the body, for both nutrition and cleansing detox purposes!

101

WATER IS THE KEY TO ALL BODY FUNCTIONS!

• Heart	• Muscles	• Energy
• Circulation	• Metabolism	• Glands
• Digestion	• Assimilation	• Sex
• Bones & Joints	• Elimination	• Nerves

Water flows through every single part of your body, cleansing and nourishing it. But the wrong kind of water, with inorganic minerals, harmful toxins, chemicals, fluorides and other contaminants can pollute and clog your body gradually stiffening it painfully. – Paul C. Bragg, N.D., Ph.D.

Pure distilled water is truly God's greatest gift to us – it is the vital natural chemistry of life, and a source of life and health. – Paul C. Bragg, N.D., Ph.D.

Why We Drink Only Pure, Distilled Water

Other than fruit and vegetable juices, my father and I would drink no other liquid except steam-produced distilled water. Today, in this polluted and poisoned world, distilled water is the purest water on the face of the earth. It contains no solid matter of any kind. It is made solely of two elements – hydrogen and oxygen. There are no minerals in it, organic or inorganic. **There is only one process that can make 100% distilled water and that is steam distillation.** In steam distillation, only pure water (H_2O) evaporates, leaving all inorganic minerals and other impurities behind.

When distilled water enters the body, it leaves no residue of any kind. It's free of salt and sodium. It's also the most perfect water to promote healthy functioning of those great "sieves," the kidneys. It's the perfect liquid for the blood. It's the ideal liquid for efficient functioning of your lungs, stomach, liver and all your miracle vital organs.

102

Let the water you drink be pure distilled water. You'll be *drinking oxygen* with this pure H_2O! As well as fresh fruit and vegetable juices – which are naturally distilled – this is a safe water to drink on our polluted planet.

Distilled Water is the #1 Health Drink

Your body is constantly working for you. Your body is 75% water (see page 110). The liquids you put in it will either nourish you or harm you, and may even eventually kill you!

Water from chemically treated public water systems – and even from many wells and springs – is likely to be loaded with poisonous chemicals and toxic trace elements. Depending upon the kinds of pipes used in the buildings, the water is likely to be overloaded with lead (from older, soldered pipe joints), zinc, copper or

---

Drinking water at correct times maximizes body effectiveness!

- 2 glasses of distilled water in morning helps activate internal organs.
- Glass of water before taking bath/shower helps lower blood pressure.
- Water 2-3 hours before bedtime, helps avoid stroke or heart attack.
- Glass of water with apple cider vinegar 30 minutes before meals, helps improve digestion, gerd and glucose levels. – Gabriel Cousens, MD

cadmium (from copper pipes). These trace elements are released in dangerous quantities by the chemical action of the water flowing against the metals of the pipes.

Your body constantly breaks down old bone and tissue cells and replaces them with new ones! As your body casts off old minerals and broken-down cells, it must obtain new supplies of essential elements in order to make healthy, new cells! (Important reason to eat healthy foods – pages 51-74.)

Scientists discovered that many disorders, including dental problems, different types of arthritis, osteoporosis and some forms of hardening of the arteries are in part due to imbalances in the levels and ratios of minerals in the body. Every body requires a proper balance of all the nutritive elements in order to remain healthy. It's as bad for a person to have too much of one item as it is to have too little of another. In order for calcium to be able to create new cells of bone and teeth, you must have adequate levels of phosphorus and magnesium. Yet, if there is too much of these minerals or too little calcium, in the diet, old bone will be taken away, but new bone will not be formed. Read more info page 67.

Although we prefer drinking distilled water, there are other clean and safe alternatives to water from your tap. You may choose to purchase water from a reputable pure water company, install a reverse osmosis machine in your home, or buy, clean water from your health food store. The key to vibrant health is to drink water that is free of chemicals and toxins.

What About Rain Water?

Even rain water – which is naturally distilled water when it leaves the clouds – is contaminated as it passes through a heavily polluted atmosphere. (Nevertheless, we love the smell of rain-washed air.) Mineral water and ground water (from springs, wells or streams) contains inorganic minerals which cannot be assimilated by the body and which can collect in the body and produce harmful deposits in the blood vessels, joints, kidneys and gallbladder. Water from reservoirs chemically treated to kill germs contains inorganic minerals and harsh chemicals (such as toxic chlorine) that are very harmful to the body!

You should know that distilled water . . .

◆ is water that's been turned into vapor so its impurities are left behind. Upon condensing, it becomes pure distilled water.

◆ is the only type of water which meets the definition of water: hydrogen + oxygen.

◆ is a perfectly natural healthy water.

◆ is also odorless, colorless and tasteless.

◆ is free of virtually all inorganic minerals, including salt.

◆ is the only natural solvent that can be taken into the body without damage to the tissues.

◆ acts as a solvent in the body by dissolving nutrients so they can be assimilated and taken into every cell.

◆ dissolves the cell wastes so the toxins can be removed.

◆ dissolves inorganic mineral substances lodged in the tissues of the body so that such substances can be eliminated in the process of purifying the body.

◆ does not leach out organic body minerals but collects and removes the toxic inorganic minerals which have been rejected by the cells and are therefore nothing more than harmful debris obstructing the normal functions of the body.

◆ is most ideal and beneficial water for all humans and animals.

◆ leaves no residue of any kind when it enters the body.

◆ is the most perfect water for the healthy functioning of those great miracle sieves, the kidneys.

◆ is the perfect liquid for the blood.

◆ is the ideal liquid for efficient functioning of the lungs, stomach, liver and all other vital organs.

◆ is universally accepted as the standard for biomedical applications and for drinking water purity.

◆ is so pure that drug prescriptions are formulated with it.

◆ is fresh, clean and pleasing to the palate.

◆ makes foods and drinks prepared with it taste noticeably better. The flavor is subtle enough not to interfere with the food it is mixed with.

◆ is the only pure water left on our polluted planet!

◆ Remember – distilled water is the healthiest water and the greatest natural water on earth!

For health's sake it's important to use only distilled water. It's a supreme internal body-cleansing agent. – Dr. Charles McFerrin, "Nature's Path"

Ten Common Sense Reasons Why We Drink Only Pure, Distilled Water

- There are over 85,000 chemicals currently used in the U.S. . . . and 500 more are being added yearly! Wherever you live, in the city or on a farm, some of these chemicals are getting into your drinking water. Beware of chemicalized water.

- No one on the face of the earth today knows what effect these chemicals could have upon the body as they blend into thousands of different combinations. It's like making a mixture of colors; just one drop could change the color.

- Proper equipment hasn't been designed yet to detect some of these toxic chemicals and may not be for years to come.

- The human body is made up of approximately 75% water (see page 110). Therefore, don't you think you should be particular about what type of water you drink?

- The U.S. Navy has been drinking distilled water for years!

- Distilled water is chemical and mineral free. Distillation removes all the chemicals and impurities from water that are possible to remove. If the distillation doesn't remove them, there is no known method today that will.

105

- The body does need minerals . . . but it is not necessary that they come from water. There is not one mineral in water which cannot be found more abundantly in food! Water is the most unreliable source of minerals because it varies from one area to another. The food we eat – not the water we drink – is the best source of organic minerals!

- Distilled water is used for intravenous feeding, inhalation therapy, prescriptions and baby formulas. Therefore, doesn't it make common sense that it's good for everyone?

- Thousands of water distillers have been sold throughout the United States and around the world to individuals, families, dentists, doctors, hospitals, nursing homes and government agencies, and these informed, alert consumers are helping protect their health by using only steam distilled water. They don't want toxic chemicals!

- With chemicals, pollutants and impurities in our water, it makes good sense to clean up the water you drink, using Mother Nature's inexpensive way – distillation.

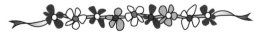

Distilled water plays a vital part in the treatment of illness, arthritis, etc.
– Dr. Allen E. Banik, author "The Choice is Clear"

Please Don't Drink Water Treated By Water Softeners!

Water softeners are being used in millions of homes because hard water is not ideal for washing your hair, clothes, dishes, etc. If you wash your hair in soft water you will discover how soft it is. ***But please do not drink the water out of water softeners!*** It's not healthy for you to drink and cook your food with because of its salt and chemical content. It contains suspended inorganic minerals and salts that produce more suds that is ideal for washing clothes and dishes; but this chemically softened water is harmful to your body.

Use distilled water for drinking and cooking to ensure a longer life and health for you and your family! You will find complete, documented reports on the web on health hazards of softened water and reasons for drinking only pure distilled water in our book, *Water – The Shocking Truth!* (See book list pages 175-178 of this book.)

At the Bragg home we use a water distiller and for our office staff we have distilled water delivered in 5 gallon bottles. Try distilled water for a year, you will see the results and never want to drink hard water again!

Keep Toxic Fluoride Out of Your Water!

Most of the water Americans drink has fluoride in it, including tap, bottled and canned drinks and foods! The ADA (American Dental Association) is insisting that the FDA (Food and Drug Association) mandate the addition of toxic fluoride to all bottled waters! Millions of innocent people have been brainwashed by the aluminum companies to erroneously believe adding sodium fluoride (their waste by-product) to drinking water will reduce tooth decay in our children. Millions of Americans drink a daily dose of sodium fluoride in their water without even knowing it.

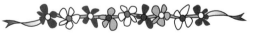

Fluoride is a waste by-product of the fertilizer and aluminum industry and it's also a Part II Poison under the UK Poisons Act 1972.

There are no regulations on fluoride content of processed foods. Many packaged foods are loaded with deadly fluoride. – Health Action Network

Fluorine is a Deadly Poison!

Sodium fluorine, a chemical "cousin" of sodium fluoride, is used as a rat and roach killer and deadly pesticide! Yet this terrible, deadly sodium fluoride, injected virtually by government, into drinking water in the proportion of 1.2 parts per million (ppm), has been declared by the United States Public Health Service to be *"absolutely safe for all human consumption."* Every qualified chemist knows that such an "absolute safety" is not only unattainable, but a total illusion!!!

Caution:
Toxic Water
Chemical Drink

Studies Show Fluoride Causes Cancer and Many Other Health Problems

- Studies show that fluoridation is causing an increase in bone cancer and deaths among males under 20.
- The growing increase in osteosarcoma is attributable to an increase in toxic fluoride.

- It is causing an increase in oral (mouth) cancer. Don't use fluoride toothpaste or allow your dentist to do fluoride treatments or use fluoride polishing paste!
- Fluoride has been linked to many health problems:
  - bone and oral cancers in humans (even in animals)
  - an ability to inhibit the DNA repair enzyme system
  - accelerates tumor growth and inhibits immune system
  - causes genetic damage in cell lines and induces melanotic tumors and fibrosarcomas.
  - other tumors/cancers strongly indicate fluoride has generalized effect of increasing them overall.
- According to study estimates, thousands of people in the United States die of cancer each year due to fluoridation of their public drinking water.

CHECK FOLLOWING WEBSITES FOR FLUORIDE UPDATES:
- www.FluorideAlert.org • fluoride.mercola.com
- www.slweb.org/bibliography.html
- www.DoctorYourself.com/carton.html

Five Hidden Toxic Dangers in Your Shower:

- **Chlorine:** Added to all municipal water supplies, this disinfectant hardens arteries, destroys proteins in the body, irritates skin and sinus conditions and aggravates any asthma, allergies and respiratory problems.

- **Chloroform:** This powerful by-product of chlorination causes excessive free radical formation (a cause of accelerated ageing!), normal cells to mutate and cholesterol to form. It's a known carcinogen!

- **DCA (Dichloroacetic acid):** This chlorine by-product alters cholesterol metabolism and has been shown to cause liver cancer in lab animals.

- **MX (toxic chlorinated acid):** Another by-product of chlorination, MX is known to cause genetic mutations that can lead to cancer growth and has been found in all chlorinated water for which it was tested.

- **Proven cause of bladder and rectal cancer:** Research proved that chlorinated water is the direct cause of 9% of all U.S. bladder cancers and 15% of all rectal cancers.

Use Shower Filter That Removes Toxins

The most effective method of removing hazards from your shower is the quick and easy installation of a filter on your shower arm. The best filter we found reduces chlorine by 95%. This shower filter also reduces iron, lead, mercury and hydrogen sulfite. Bacterial, fungal and mildew growth are also effectively inhibited. It has a 12-18 month filter life-span and you can easily clean the filter by backwashing and replace only when needed. I have been using an approved shower filter for many years and really enjoy my chlorine-free showers!

Start enjoying safe, chlorine-free showers right away. It's essential to reducing your risk of heart disease and cancer and to ease the strain on your immune system. You may even get rid of long-standing conditions – from sinus and respiratory problems to dry, itchy skin.

"Water contains healing; it is the simplest, cheapest and – if used correctly – the safest remedy. Water is my best friend and will remain all my life!"
– Father Sebastian Kneipp, Father of Hydrotherapy • www.Kneipp.com

You Get More Toxic Exposure from Taking a Chlorinated Water Shower Than From Drinking the Same Water!

Two of the very highly toxic and volatile chemicals, trichloroethylene and chloroform, have been proven as toxic contaminants found in most all municipal drinking U.S. water supplies. The National Academy of Sciences has estimated that hundreds of people die in the United States each year from the cancers caused largely by ingesting water pollutants from inhalation as air pollutants in the home. Inhalation exposure to water pollutants is largely ignored. Recent shocking data indicates that hot showers can liberate about 50% of the chloroform and 80% of the trichloroethylene into the air.

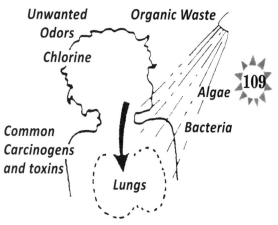

Tests show your body can absorb more toxic chlorine from a 10 minute shower than drinking 8 glasses of the same water. How can that be? A warm shower opens up your pores, causing your skin to act like a sponge. As a result, you not only inhale the toxic chlorine vapors, you absorb them through your skin, directly into your bloodstream – at a toxic rate that is up to 6 times higher than drinking it.

In terms of cumulative damage to your health, showering in chlorinated water is one of the most dangerous risks you take daily. Short-term risks include: eyes, sinus, throat, skin and lung irritation. Long-term risks include: excessive free radical formation (that ages you!), higher vulnerability to genetic mutation and cancer development; and difficulty metabolizing cholesterol that can cause hardened arteries. – Science News

---

ACV SHOWER MASSAGE GIVES EXTRA BODY BONUS: (in 32oz. bottle dilute 1/2 cup apple cider vinegar and water.) Pour all over body before you get out of shower. Now take thick washcloth, rub in for 3-5 minutes. When drying rub thick dry washcloth over back and then front too. Feels so good! – PB

THE 75% WATERY HUMAN

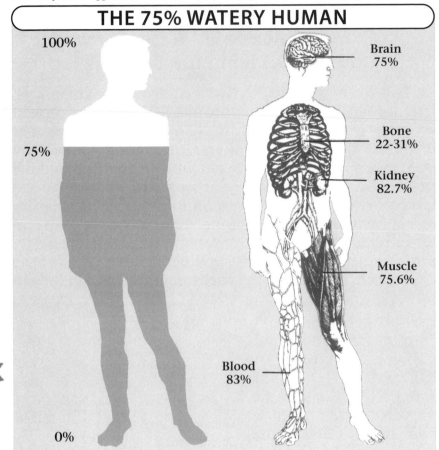

100%

75%

75%

0%

Brain
75%

Bone
22-31%

Kidney
82.7%

Muscle
75.6%

Blood
83%

110

The amount of water in human body, averaging 75%, varies considerably even from one part of the body to another area as shown here. A lean man may hold 75% of his weight in body water, while a woman – because of her larger proportion of adipose tissues – may be only 52% water. The lowering of the water content in the blood is what triggers the hypothalamus, the brain's vital thirst center, to send out its familiar urgent demand for a drink of water! Please obey and drink ample amounts (8 glasses) of purified, distilled water daily. By the time you feel thirsty, you're already dehydrated. – American Running & Fitness Association

WATER PERCENTAGE IN VARIOUS BODY PARTS:

Teeth	10%	Spleen	75.5%
Bones	22-31%	Lungs	80%
Cartilage	55%	Blood	83%
Red blood corpuscles	68.7%	Bile	86%
Liver	71.5%	Plasma	90%
Brain	75%	Lymph	94%
Muscle tissue	75%	Saliva	95.5%

This chart shows why 8-10 glasses of pure water daily is so important.

You Must Give Your Body Gentle Sunshine

The Importance of Healing Sunshine

Doctor Sunshine's speciality is heliotherapy. His great prescription is solar energy. Each tiny blade of grass, every vine, tree, bush, flower, fruit and vegetable draws its life from solar energy. All living things on earth depend on solar energy for their very existence. This earth would be a barren, frigid place if it were not for the magic rays of the sun. The sun gives us light . . . and were it not for light, there would be no you or me!

People who are denied the vital miracle rays of the sun have a pallid look. They are actually dying for the want of solar energy! Weak, ailing, anemic people may be sun-starved and, in our opinion, many people are sick simply because they are starving for gentle sunshine.

111

Enjoy Sunshine For Super Health

That is why my father and I have always loved precious sunshine. That's why we made our main home in California, the golden sunshine state. We have an organic farm in Santa Barbara near the ocean where we get the benefits of the clean air and miracle sunshine. Seek fresh, clean air, gentle sunshine and organic sun-kissed foods, then soon super health will leap out and be yours to treasure throughout a long, youthful, productive, happy life!

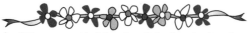

Sunshine Vitamin D3 – essential for health. Analysis of more that 15,000 Americans, with low blood levels of Vitamin D3, were 30% more likely to have high blood pressure, 40% more apt to have high triglycerides, 98% more likely to be diabetic and 129% more apt to be obese. Researchers noted that low Vitamin D3 may also be a culprit for Fibromyalgia, Multiple Sclerosis, Rheumatoid Arthritis and other joint diseases.

 The sun does not shine for a few trees and flowers, but for the whole world's joy. – Henry Ward Beecher

Doctor Healing Sunshine Saved Bragg's Life!

We believe that the Alpine sunshine – at an altitude of 5,000 feet in the Swiss Alps played a tremendous part in my father's miracle recovery from tuberculosis. When my father was diagnosed with tuberculosis at 16, three TB Sanitariums later, the best TB doctors in USA declared his case *hopeless and incurable!* Yet he was led to Dr. August Rollier of Leysin, Switzerland, the greatest living authority on heliotherapy (sun cure). High in the Swiss Alps, Dad's sick and wasted body was exposed to the gentle healing rays of the sun and was fed an abundance of natural, sun-ripened foods.

Dad's introduction to sunbathing was supervised very closely. My father's first day in the alpine sun he only exposed his feet! Each day thereafter the doctor instructed him to expose more of his body to the direct gentle rays of the sun. The conditioning period to expose his body to the sunshine extended over a period of weeks. By then his body was conditioned to more gentle sunshine.

The doctor believed the best healing rays of the sun were in the early morning and late afternoon. Dad would start his sunbathing program as early as 7 a.m. and enjoy the early sun rays. In the cool morning the healing rays were at their highest point. By 11 a.m. they began to disappear and hot infrared rays took over. This was the time Dr. Rollier advised his patients not to sunbathe! Then after 3 p.m. they were again allowed to expose their bodies to the gentle rays that had now returned as the hot infrared rays subsided.

A healing miracle happened. In just two years he was transformed into a vitally strong young man who radiated health! Throughout Paul Bragg's long, fulfilled life he was healthy, happy, powerful in sports and always enjoyed the great outdoors and the healing rays of the gentle sun on his body.

Gentle Sunbathing Works Miracles!

When you begin sunbathing, start with short time periods until you condition your body to take more. The best time for beginners to start taking 10 and 15 minute sunbaths is in the early morning sunshine until 10 a.m. or late afternoon sunshine after 3 p.m. Between 11 and 3 we usually avoid stronger, burning rays. Please don't use sunscreens with PABA; the chemicals are harmful.

The cool rays of the sun rejuvenate the skin and help keep your eyes healthy and in focus. You will find that as you detoxify your body and eliminate toxins, you will be able to develop a beautiful natural tan and healthy glow. The gentle sun is a tonic for frazzled nerves. Its cool rays calm, quiet and soothe the nerves while helping to promote a relaxed feeling. You can combine a nap with a sunbath, wherein you will help refill the body reservoirs with Nerve Force. After gently sunning, pat on some organic apple cider vinegar (undiluted).

Gentle Sunshine – The Great Healer

The rays of the sun are powerful germicides! As the skin soaks up more of these rays, it stores enormous amounts of this germ-killing energy and vitamin D (see pages 114-116). The sun provides one of the finest remedies for the nervous person who suffers from anxiety, worry, frustration and stresses. When these tense people lie in the gentle sunshine, its powerful rays provide them with the relaxation that their nerves and bodies need!

As you bask in the warm, gentle sunshine (not the hot midday/afternoon sun), millions of nerve endings absorb the solar energy (*rich in vitamin D*) and transfer it to your body's nervous system. Gentle sunshine is a soothing tonic, a stimulant and above all, a Great Healer!

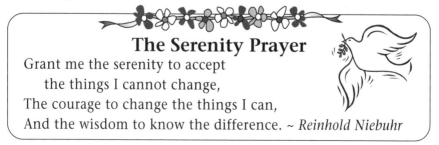

The Serenity Prayer

Grant me the serenity to accept
   the things I cannot change,
The courage to change the things I can,
And the wisdom to know the difference. ~ *Reinhold Niebuhr*

Chlorophyll is Miracle Liquid Sunshine

Perform this experiment to determine the value of sunshine in the matter of life and death. Find a beautiful lawn, where the grass is like a green carpet. Cover up a small space of that beautiful lawn with a piece of wood or a small box. Day by day you will soon notice that the beautiful grass that once was full of plant blood, precious chlorophyll, will fade and turn a sickly yellow. Tragically, it withers and dies – death by sun starvation!

Eat Healthy Sun-Ripened Foods

The same thing happens to your body when deprived of life-giving sun rays, or when you fail to eat enough sun-cooked foods such as ripe juicy fruits and vegetables. We must have direct sun rays on our bodies and at least 60% of food we eat must have been ripened by the sun's rays! Eat fresh fruits and vegetables. When we eat them, we absorb chlorophyll, the rich, nourishing blood of the plant. Chlorophyll is the pure, distilled solar energy that the plant has absorbed from the sun, and is the richest and most nourishing food you can put into your body! **"Chlorophyll is liquid sunshine!"** Green plants alone possess the secret of how to capture this powerful solar energy and pass it on to man and every living creature. When you take in gentle sunshine on the outside of your body while inside your body you consume 60%-70% organic raw fruits and vegetables, you will soon glow with radiant health!

Vitamin D3 – The Sunshine Vitamin

Your body is designed to get the vitamin D it needs by producing it when your skin is exposed to sunlight. The part of the sun's rays that is important is ultraviolet B (UVB). This is the most natural way to get vitamin D.

Small amounts of gentle sunlight on your skin cells causes them to manufacture vitamin D3. Even as little as 10-15 minutes, 2 to 3 times a week should be enough. Sunscreen can reduce or even shut down the synthesis of vitamin D3, so we recommend exposure to gentle early morning or late afternoon rays without use of sunscreen.

Sunshine Vitamin D3 – Essential for Health

Vital vitamin D3 helps the body utilize calcium and phosphorus to build bones and teeth. Vitamin D3 also helps the skin heal and boosts your immune system. Statistics from a California survey of American women found those women with higher sun exposure and those with a high dietary intake of vitamin D3, had a lower risk of breast cancer. Evidence also points to a link between vitamin D3 and reduced risk of colon cancer and bone fractures.

An analysis of more than 15,000 Americans, those with low blood levels of Vitamin D3, were 30% more likely to have high blood pressure, 40% more apt to have high triglycerides, 98% more likely to be diabetic and 129% more apt to be obese. Researchers noted that low Vitamin D3 may also be a culprit for Fibromyalgia, Multiple Sclerosis, Rheumatoid Arthritis and other joint diseases.

Five Ways Vitamin D3 Can Save Your Life

1. **Reduces Risk of Heart Disease:** Vitamin D3 improves blood flow by relaxing the blood vessels and lowering blood pressure.

2. **Promotes Weight Loss:** You need Vitamin D3 to effectively help you lose weight. Your insulin works better and Vitamin D3 helps you lose belly fat. Diabetes is also related to low Vitamin D3 levels.

3. **Supports Immune System:** Gentle sunlight increases production of the white blood cells (lymphocytes and gamma globulin), which increases the body's defense mechanism to fight against infections.

4. **Fewer Bone Fractures:** Without Vitamin D3, calcium can't be absorbed. But if you get enough vitamin D3, it helps you avoid osteoporosis, bone fractures and falling, which is a cause of morbidity among elderly.

5. **Reduces Risk of Cancers:** Sunshine Vitamin D3, may prevent certain types of cancer – breast, colon, ovaries, lung and prostate. A deficiency in Vitamin D3 is one of the main causes for the incidence of such cancers.

Sunshine gives energy and life to the earth, to all plants, trees and all living creatures.

How Much Vitamin D3 is Necessary?

There is evidence supporting the near-miraculous healing power of Vitamin D3. People under 50 years need 1,000 IUs, 50-70 years need 2,000 IUs and those over 70 need 2,000-5,000 IUs of vitamin D3 daily, more in special cases. Older people's ability to produce vitamin D3 from sunlight declines. That's why it's important for those over 70 to get vitamin D3 from supplements and foods: wheat germ, raw sunflower seeds, cod liver oil, sweet potatoes, corn bread, eggs, alfalfa, saltwater fish, sardines, salmon, tuna, liver and natural vegetable oils are good sources of vitamin D3 (see web: *www.doctoroz.com*).

Five Ways To Get Vitamin D3

1. **15 minutes of high-noon sun exposure** in warmer climates few times a week. *(We prefer early or late sun.)*
2. **Fatty Fish and Cod Liver Oil:** If you have been warned to stay out of the sun, another good source Vitamin D3 is oily fish, such as salmon, tuna, mackerel and trout.
3. **Fortified Dairy Products** *(We prefer non-dairy.)*
4. **Multi-Vitamin Supplements:** Most all multi-vitamins have a substantial amount of vitamin D3.
5. **Vitamin D3 Supplements:** 1000 to 2000 IUs Vitamin D3 recommended daily. *(Seniors 2000 to 3000 IUs.)*

Taken from: "Good Morning America's" Medical Contributor
Marie Savard – abcnews.go.com/GMA

Vitamin D3 is made when UVB light from the sun is absorbed by the skin. This is most natural form. Most supplements sold today are Vitamin D3 (animal source – lanolin) or Vitamin D2 (yeast derived) ideal for vegetarians and vegans. Vitamin D3 is a more potent form of Vitamin D and has a better stable shelf-life. Learn more by reading "Vitamin D Solution" by Michael F. Holick, Ph.D., M.D., Professor Boston University and recipient of prestigious "Linus Pauling Prize" for his extensive research on Vitamin D.

Morning light helps best in regulation of your body's circadian rhythm and energy balance. Circadian rhythm is the body's physical, mental and behavioral changes that follow a roughly 24-hour cycle.

We all grow healthier in nature, gentle sunshine and love!

Chapter 10

You Must Give Your Body Rest

Don't Overwork, Stress or Burden Your Body

Doctor Rest is another health specialist always at your command to help you achieve Supreme Vitality and Health! We believe the word *rest* is the most misunderstood word in the English language. Some people's idea of resting is to sit down and drink a cup of a strong stimulant such as coffee, black tea or caffeinated soft drinks. This is typified by the *coffee break*. To us, rest means repose, freedom from activity and quiet tranquility. It means peace of mind and spirit. It means to rest without anxiety or worry! Rest means to refresh and should renew your whole nervous system and your entire body – physically, mentally, and spiritually.

To rest means to allow free circulation (no restrictions) of blood throughout the body, which is important for health. The best rest can only be secured when your body is relaxed and freed from restrictive clothing. Your clothes should be comfortably loose. Are your shoes too tight? Your collar? Your hat? Your stockings? Your watch, belt, undergarments, bra*? If yes, then you're not resting!

117

Allow Muscles and Nerves to Relax

Why do we rest? You often hear people say, *"I must take a break!"* The art of resting is something that must be acquired and concentrated upon! Muscles that are tense may be uncomfortable, but if you move them you will only prolong their discomfort. Permit them to relax and the distress should disappear within 15 minutes.

*Please read "Dressed To Kill" by S. Singer
on breast cancer and bra studies.*

*Women, please cut wires out of bras that hinder your circulation.
I prefer not to wear a bra but instead a loose chemise. – Patricia Bragg*

Enjoy Rest and Naps –
It's Not a Crime to Relax!

In order to rest and nap, you must learn to clear your mind of all anxiety, worries and emotional problems. When the muscles and nerves are relaxed, the heart action slows – especially when you take long, slow, deep breaths. This will help promote a deeper relaxation and more peaceful rest that promotes more total health! The greatest place to rest, relax and renew your body's Vital Force is under the blue sky, in the clean, fresh air. On hot summer days, enjoy the cool shade of trees.

Tension and Relaxation
Create the Heartbeat of Life

As you obey and live by the Laws of Mother Nature you'll automatically earn the right to relax when your body needs relaxation. There is nothing wrong with tension. Tension is part of life. For example – when we walk out onto the platform to lecture before 5,000 people for 2 hours we are bound to feel some tension! Life is movement and movement requires tension as well as release. How is that fact expressed in your body?

Say Good-Bye to Tiredness – Hello Super Energy

- Sit down and kick off your shoes. Let tiredness go away and now relax!

- Now start breathing in, easily and deeply, then breathe out tiredness. Next breathe deeply in a feeling of complete peace and relaxation.

- Curl your toes down tight, now relax toes and feet. Repeat exercise: Now tighten, then relax fingers and slowly do arms, legs, butt, etc.

- Breathe out slowly all the pressures, stress and tiredness of the day. Then breathe in refreshing joy, health, love and peace.

- Now relax, close eyes for 10 minutes, then afterwards stand up and stretch.

- Stand, stretch arms up, now do wide windmill circles, then reverse circles.

- Now stretch your body, arms and legs – sideways, up and down, etc.

Nervous Tension can ruin your health in dozens of ways and diminish your productivity and even shorten your lifespan.
– Dr. Edmund Jacobson, author of "You Must Relax"

You have a miraculous muscle in your chest cavity that is active from the moment it begins to function before birth to the instant of your death. That miracle muscle is your heart. How does it keep going for so many years? Study it closely. Observe exactly how it works. It tenses and then relaxes, tenses and relaxes. Thus it can go on and on and on. There is a great lesson for us here.

The heart is like life itself. It should be made up of tension and relaxation. To get a task done – whether it is large or small – we must draw upon our Nerve Force reserves. We put an extra push into our efforts and this extra push is tension. If our nerves are healthy and we are working correctly, when the effort of the task is over we should automatically have the feeling of relaxation.

You can't force relaxation any more than you can change the beating of your heart. Relaxation is a feeling, always remember that. It is something that works naturally within your nervous system. Live by Mother Nature's Laws and you will never have to worry about relaxation. This feeling will come to you naturally.

Relaxation is a Healthy, Soothing Feeling

There is no other way to express it. This feeling is not something you can turn off and on at will. It is something that must be built up in the conscious and the subconscious mind, something you build up in every one of the billions of cells in your body, in your entire nervous system, in your vital organs and in your muscles.

Relaxation is a feeling. Your feelings allow your nerves to relax. Your feelings can banish stress, strain and tensions to bring calm, inner peace and serenity. Feeling is the life force within you that is always working for you. All it needs is a chance. It is astonishing how few people get their physical, mental and emotional debris out of the way and let feeling work for them.

Nothing in all creation is so like God as stillness. – Meister Eckhart

Peace is not a season, it is an important way for a healthy life!

Mother Nature Knows What's Best!

Let health, air, sun and complete rest work for you. With a serene clear eye and confidence, put yourself in Mother Nature's hands. Let her run your machine, heal your hurts and comfort you in sickness and adversity. Make Mother Nature your partner and – when you are resting, relaxing, and recreating new energy – she will always be there with her loving hand on your shoulder. So be a child of Mother Nature. Don't look for sophisticated thrills, but find your joy and diversion in relaxation, reading, fun, friends, exercise and other pursuits that are simple, down to earth and are at one with Mother Nature. Your rewards will be many – including renewed health – physically, mentally and spiritually and a new awareness of the great out of doors she gives us so generously to enjoy.

As you obey and live by the Laws of Mother Nature (see page 49) you will automatically earn the right to relax when your body needs relaxation. One of the predominant suggestions of this book is a gradual return to Mother Nature and her natural way of living. In food, breathing, rest, exercise, sunshine, fasting and a simplicity in living habits, try to reach a nearness to Mother Nature that makes you almost one with her.

Begin to live as Mother Nature wants you to live. Seek to feel that she claims you and you are part of all healthy, growing things. Put yourself into her hands and let her guide you! You will rekindle your own youth in the quiet beauty of a hill or meadow. If you are to grow more healthy and youthful, begin by believing you can and that Mother Nature is eager to aid you! If you are a prisoner of the city, make it a point to get out to the parks or country or the seashore where you can really find true rest, tranquillity and serenity. By living in simplicity and purity, you will be filled with more peace, joy and love.

There is no biological reason why human beings should not reach the age of 150.
– Dr. Alexis Carrel, Pioneer Scientist, The Rockefeller Institute

When your body is completely relaxed then you will experience an inner peace, inner serenity and the true joy of living.

Be good to your body and it will be good to you! Live so that the feeling of relaxation will come to you when it is needed. Be a friend to yourself! Treat yourself right so you can enjoy a long, healthy and relaxed life. The kingdom of heaven is within.

Plan, plot and follow through so you have time for rest, recreation, exercise and a good night's sleep. You can't get a good night's sleep if you overload your stomach and nervous system! Your body will have a good night's sleep if you have some vigorous exercise, plenty of fresh air, quiet and gentle sunlight. Have a balanced program of living then let Mother Nature do the rest.

Good Sleep is Cornerstone of Good Health

Eight hours nightly is the optimal amount of sleep for most adults! Science has established that a sleep deficit can have serious, far reaching effects on your health!

Interrupted or Lack of Proper Sleep Can:

- Dramatically weaken your immune system
- Accelerate tumor growth with severe sleep dysfunctions
- Cause a pre-diabetic state, making you feel hungry and then you over fuel your body causing obesity
- Seriously impair your memory. Even a single night of poor sleep (4-6 hours) can impact ability to think clearly
- Impair your performance on physical or mental tasks
- Can also increase stress-related disorders including: heart disease, stomach ulcers, constipation, mood disorders, personality upsets and depression

Healthful Tips for Sound, Recharging Sleep
Excerpts from Dr. Mercola – www.mercola.com

The good news is there are many natural techniques you can learn to restore your "sleep health" (don't take sleeping pills). Whether you have difficulty falling asleep or feel inadequately rested when waking up, you can find some relief from the tips on the next 2 pages.

Relaxation is a beautiful soothing feeling within your body and mind.

Health Tips for Sound Recharging Sleep

• **Sleep in complete darkness.** Even the tiniest bit of light in the room can disrupt your internal clock and your pineal gland's production of melatonin and serotonin. Little bits of light pass directly through your optic nerve to your hypothalamus, which controls your biological clock. Light signals your brain that it's time to wake up and start preparing your body for ACTION!!!

• **Wear an eye mask to block out light.** It is not always easy to block out every stream of light using curtains or blinds.

• **Keep your bedroom at a lower temperature 60-65°F is best for sleeping.** Scientists believe a cooler bedroom is most conducive to sleep since it mimics the body's natural temperature drop.

• **Check bedroom for Electro-Magnetic Fields (EMFs).** EMF's can disrupt the pineal gland and production of melatonin and serotonin. To do this you will need a gauss meter. Before bed unplug any phones or electronics near the bed, even when staying in hotels!

• **Move alarm clocks and other electric devices away from bed.** It adds worry when you stare at it all night – 2 am, 3 am, 4:30 am. Prior to electricity, people would go to bed shortly after sundown and rise with the sun as most animals do. Mother Nature intended this for humans as well.

• **Get to bed as early as possible.** Your body recharges between the hours of 11 pm and 1 am. Also, your gallbladder dumps toxins during this same period. If you are awake, the toxins back up into your liver, which can further disrupt your sleep and your health.

• **Establish a good bedtime routine.** This could be meditation, deep breathing, aromatherapy, essential oils or a massage.

Aromatherapy – A Healer For Centuries

Aromatherapy is the practice of using natural oils extracted from flowers, leaves, bark or other parts of a plant to enhance psychological and physical well-being. The inhaled aroma from these "essential" oils is widely believed to stimulate brain function. Essential oils can also be absorbed through the skin, where they travel through the bloodstream and can promote whole-body healing. Aromatherapy has the power to work miracles, to uplift and heal. Treat yourself to the delights and fragrances of essential oils. Smelling beautiful roses, flowers and fruit blossoms is also recharging.
See more info on Aromatherapy page 163. – *www.Aromatherapy.com*

- **It is best not to drink fluids two hours before bedtime.** This helps reduce the likelihood or lessens frequency of needing to use the bathroom at night. Also make sure that you empty the bladder right before you go to bed.
- **Have a high-protein drink/shake several hours before bed.** This helps provide L-tryptophan needed for your melatonin and serotonin production (SlimFast, Ensure).
- **Avoid before-bed snacks, particularly grains and sugars.**
- **Take a hot bath, shower or sauna before bed.** The temperature drop from getting out of the bath or shower helps to signal your body it's time for bed and sleep.
- **Wear socks to bed.** Study shows wearing socks reduces night wakings. You could put hot water in a glass bottle near your feet at night. It's so comforting!
- **Put work away at least one hour before bed.** This gives your mind a chance to unwind so you can go to sleep feeling calm, not hyped up or anxious about tomorrow's deadlines.
- **No TV one hour before bed.** TV disrupts your pineal gland function.
- **Keep a Daily Journal.** (See page 74). Write in the morning when your brain is functioning at its peak and cortisol levels are high.

Lifestyle Suggestions That Enhance Sleep

- **Avoid stimulants:** caffeine (in coffee, some teas, even green teas, soft drinks, chocolate, sugar) and nicotine (found in cigarettes and other tobacco products).
- **Don't drink alcohol** to "help" you sleep.
- **Have herbal teas** – anise, lemon balm, *Sleepytime*, chamomile (beware some green teas have caffeine), or try melatonin, tryptophan (5HTP), valerian, calcium and magnesium supplements; they work miracles.
- **Exercise regularly**, but try to be finished with your workout no sooner than 2 hours prior to bedtime.
- **Avoid foods you may be sensitive to.** Reactions can cause excess congestion, gastrointestinal upset, bloating or gas.
- **Associate your bed with recharging sleep** – it's wise not to sit on it to work or watch TV. *Try a memory 2" foam topper (so comfortable) on your firm mattress.*
- **Don't nap during the day**, if you suffer from insomnia. Remember, earn better sleep by exercise and day activity.

The Lord gives strength to those who are weary. – Isaiah 40:29

Get Peaceful Sleep – Stop Snoring

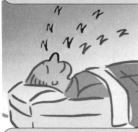 If snoring is happening frequently it can affect the quantity and quality of your sleep and that of family members. Snoring can lead to poor sleep, daytime fatigue, irritability, and increased health problems.

Bedtime Remedies To Help You Stop Snoring

Clear nasal passages. Having a stuffy nose makes inhalation difficult and 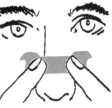 creates a vacuum in your throat, which can lead to snoring. Clear passages naturally with nasal strips (*BreatheRight.com*) or a Breathing Detox (see below) to help you breathe more easily while sleeping.

Somnoplasty: An Effective Treatment For Blocked Nasal Airways and Snoring

Somnoplasty is a minimally invasive procedure that can be performed as an in-office surgery. It is done under local anesthesia with typical time lasting 15-20 minutes. The procedure involves using radio frequency heat to shrink relevant tissues leading to the shrinkage of inner tissues. For chronic nasal obstruction – the turbinates are targeted; habitual snoring the soft palate and uvula; and sleep apnea the base of the tongue and other airway structures.

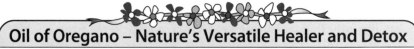

Oil of Oregano – Nature's Versatile Healer and Detox

Oil of Oregano is a powerful herbal body defender and cleanser and is used to fight: viruses; flus; colds; allergies; asthma; E. coli; Salmonella; parasitic yeast and bacterial infections; upset stomach; menstrual problems; urinary tract problems and arthritis. Take with food. Available in capsules or drops at health and vitamin stores. When needed for winter cold maintenance do the following Breathing Detox:

Breathing Detox: Place 2-3 drops of "Oil of Oregano" in 2 qts. boiling water. Put towel over head, breathe in vapors through mouth, then nose. It's powerful, keep your eyes closed! This opens up lungs to remove congestion. Relieves colds, flu, bronchitis congestion. Do as needed 1-3 times daily.

Each patient carries his own doctor inside him. – Albert Schweitzer, M.D.

Stress Reducing Guidelines:

Avoid the super-person complex! Some people want too much from themselves. They are perfectionists. They are full of tensions from pushing themselves beyond their human capacity to perform. One person cannot be skilled in everything. Do your best with those tasks which you cannot do so well and let it go at that. No one asks or expects you to accomplish the impossible, so don't demand it of yourself! You will have a much longer, healthier and happier life.

Talk out your worries! Don't bottle everything up. If you feel you have a legitimate "beef" against someone, go to that person and quietly talk things out. Just as it takes a good storm to clear up the atmosphere when the weather is "tense," a good talk will usually clear up a disturbed emotional atmosphere. Do not harbor resentments! Get them off your chest quickly and as calmly as possible! Nine times out of ten they arise from a misunderstanding – either on your part, the other person's or both.

125

This applies to all relationships – whether it be your mate, children, in-laws, relatives, friends or your co-workers, etc. So many husbands and wives or parents and children have let resentments build up inside until they can no longer communicate with one another. You may need to place your confidence in a good friend, therapist, relative or clergy person. Talking things over with someone who can be objective will relieve stress and enable you to view your plight in a clear light and help you find a logical solution to your worry or problem.

Beware of your temper. Temper is too good of a thing to lose! Under control, your temper becomes a driving force that can push you forward to the accomplishment of worthwhile goals. Out of control, your temper can destroy you, your relationships, your business and others as well. When you get irate you are throwing away precious nerve energy. A "fit of temper" often causes nervous and physical exhaustion.

The greatest discovery of my generation is that human beings can alter their lives by altering their attitudes of mind. – William James (1842-1920)

Start counting and keep on counting when you feel your temper rising. Don't say anything you will regret! Get into some vigorous physical activity at once. The best way to cool your anger is to take a brisk walk in the open air. Get away from the person or situation that is sending you into a rage. Swimming, gardening, housework or any other type of physical work or exercise will help work off your temper constructively.

It's Important To Live Joyously with Yourself

Remember you came into this world alone and you will leave it alone. It's nice to have a good family, friends and a mate, but – above all – you must learn to love living with yourself! Maintain a high personal dignity level, even with yourself. You must be good company for yourself. We have never been bored in our lives. We go on long hikes and get to understand ourselves better. As we grow to understand ourselves better, we get to understand other people more.

Lead a busy, happy, creative life. You will have a happy, well-rounded, balanced day with your meditation and prayer, your exercises and deep breathing, healthy eating program and reading new, instructive books, plus continuing with your daily work. A busy person is a happy person with little time to worry. Life becomes a great adventure. Enjoy every minute of it! We get 24 precious hours a day. So live each day as though it were your last!

Have an Attitude of Gratitude!

Gratitude creates happiness because it makes us feel full and complete. Gratitude is the realization that we have everything we need. One of the truths about gratitude is that it is impossible to feel both the positive emotion of thankfulness and a negative emotion such as anger or fear at the same time. Gratitude gives only positive feelings – love, compassion, joy, and hope. As we focus on what we are thankful for, fear, anger, and bitterness simply melt away.*

Excerpt from "Attitudes of Gratitude" by M.J. Ryan

Ten Great Stress Busters & Mood Builders:

1. Turn on your favorite music and dance.
2. Enroll in a yoga class, or take tai chi, Qi gong, Pilates or stretching class.
3. Call a good friend and have some laughs.
4. Read inspiring Bragg books and health magazines.
5. Take a hot herbal bubble bath or vinegar bath.
6. Go to the gym or take a brisk fresh air walk.
7. Get a massage – best at home when possible.
8. Write and release your feelings in daily journal.
9. Watch an inspiring movie, comedy or travelogue.
10. Close your eyes, relax, do 'yoga breathing' – breathe in slowly through nose, letting air fill lungs completely down to diaphragm. Hold in briefly, then exhale through mouth slowly.

Enjoy Life – Slow Down

Life has lots of simple things to enjoy. But if you move too fast, you might overlook them. Don't be in such a hurry. Look at the world around you. Notice the grass, the flowers, the sunrise or sunset – Mother Nature is all around you. Take time to pause and reflect.

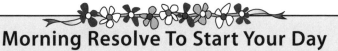

Morning Resolve To Start Your Day

I will this day live a simple, sincere and serene life; repelling promptly every thought of impurity, discontent, anxiety, fear, and discouragement. I will cultivate health, cheerfulness, happiness, charity and the love of brotherhood; exercising economy in expenditure, generosity in giving, carefulness in conversation and diligence in appointed service. I will be faithful in those habits of prayer, study, work, nutrition, physical exercise, deep breathing and good posture. I shall fast for 24 hours each week, eat only healthy foods and get sufficient sleep each night. I will make every effort to improve myself – physically, mentally, emotionally and spiritually every day.

– *Morning prayer used by Patricia Bragg and her father, Paul Bragg*

Decades of Amazement as Life Rolls By

Where did our years go? They went by so fast.
When we're young they seem to cra-a-wl,
With each decade, they fly past!

At 29 we're the center; At 30 we feel supreme
But 40 strikes terror; Life's not what it seems.
By 50 we've reached maturity; At 60 we accept seniority.
When we're filled with excitement of creative living,
There's no room for depression and despair!

But at 65, wisdom that comes from experience
Then takes over and we learn to accept ourselves as we are.
Each new day is a gift to be treasured,
Enabling us to go far!

At 75, life is for the living
But it is through our sharing, loving and giving
that we reach the Stars of Joy, Peace
and the Possibilities of Eternity!

128

– by Ruth Lubin, who started writing poetry and sculpturing at 80!
PS: Ruth has been a fan of the Bragg Healthy Lifestyle for over 58 years!

PROMISE YOURSELF . . .

To be so strong that nothing can disturb your peace of mind.

To talk health, happiness and prosperity to every person you meet.

To make all your friends feel that there is something in them.

To look at the sunny side of everything and make your optimism come true.

To think only the best, to work only for the best, and to expect only the best.

To be just as enthusiastic about the success of others as you are about your own.

To forget the mistakes of the past and press on to the greater achievements of the future.

To wear a cheerful countenance at all times and give every living creature you meet a smile.

To give so much time to the improvement of yourself that you have no time to criticize others.

To be too large for worry, too noble for anger, too strong for fear and too happy to permit the presence of trouble.

To think well of yourself and to proclaim this fact to the world, not in loud words but great deeds.

To life in faith that the whole world is on your side so long as you are true to the best that is in you.

– Christian D. Larson
Author & Influential Leader

Chapter 11

You Must Keep Your Body Clean – Inside & Out

Your Tongue Never Lies

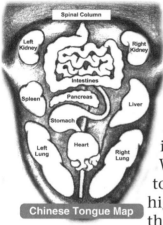

Chinese Tongue Map

The tongue should be called *"the Magic Mirror."* The tongue, a spongy organ reveals the great amount of toxic waste poison stored throughout the body. One means a doctor uses to diagnose a person is to say, *"Let me see your tongue."* When the doctor sees a white-coated tongue, he knows that person is in a highly toxic condition. This is one of the oldest methods of diagnosis used by health professionals around the world. Remember that the tongue is one end of a tube that averages 30 feet in length, extending from your mouth to the anus. When the tongue is coated, it shows that Mother Nature is trying to push out some of the deep buried toxic waste in the body. A water fast helps your garbage miracle workers dig out and then flush out the toxins! Fasting performs miracles!

129

Sick people often have a heavily coated tongue, plus bad breath. While fasting or adhering to a strict fruit diet, such as apples and oranges you will notice that the tongue becomes coated. The fasting and the fruit diet starts to loosen the stored filthy toxic body poisons. **The tongue is "the Magic Mirror" of the stomach, and the entire mucus membrane system.**

You should cleanse your tongue by gently scraping its surface with the round tip of a spoon or tongue scraper. Begin at back of your tongue. Gently press down and pull the spoon forward towards your tongue's tip; repeat as necessary until the entire top of your tongue has been cleaned of its toxic coating. The toxins scraped show one of your immediate *fast* results.

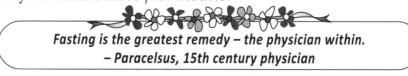

Fasting is the greatest remedy – the physician within.
– Paracelsus, 15th century physician

Daily Tongue Brushing is a Good Habit

After scraping your tongue, use your toothbrush to lightly brush your tongue from the back to the tip (it's a good habit to brush tongue daily). Then you should gargle with a mixture of 1 teaspoon of organic raw apple cider vinegar in ½ glass of water to rinse any remaining germs or toxins from your mouth. Repeat this cleansing 1 - 2 times daily during a detox water fast or a beginners juice fast (also try Oil Pulling, see page 131). Your body will continue to push toxic slime out through the tongue! This tongue coating shows you are doing deep cleansing. It's an accurate indication of the amount of mucus and other toxic poisons stored in the tissues that are now being eliminated from the inside surfaces of the stomach, intestines and your entire body. (*Also try skin brushing, see page 161.*)

You can now see by the coated tongue how much toxic poison you have stored in your body. The tongue's surface reveals the great amount of encumbrances that have been clogging up your body because of unhealthy living and the eating of refined, high-fat, sugar, salt, meat and dairy toxic-forming foods.

The Human Pipe System Must Be Kept Clean and Healthy

The entire human pipe system, especially the microscopically small capillaries (the smallest pipes in the body, about the size of a human hair), become "chronically" clogged by the heavily processed, foodless foods of civilization. There are no special diets that can clean a dirty, heavily coated tongue. Your body is self-cleansing and self-healing when you give it a chance!

To be well, stay well and to be free from aches and pains, you must live each day so that you eliminate the toxic poisons you have accumulated over the years.

Eat to live, and not live to eat. Many dishes, many diseases.
– Benjamin Franklin, 1706-1790

Prevention is always preferable to the cure.

The Toxicless Diet, Body Purification and Healing System calls for large amounts of organic raw and lightly cooked vegetables and fresh fruits; weekly 24-hour fasts and periodic fasts lasting from 3 to 10 days. We know what miracles this System of Internal Purification can do for the sick and prematurely old person. So did Professor A. E. Crews of Edinburgh University – who had performed extensive dietary restriction experiments on both mammals and worms – noted on page 134.

We faithfully fast 24 hours every Monday and the first 3 days of each month. We never worry about being overweight – our weight remains balanced and normal! Wait until you experience this miraculous cleansing process! You will greatly benefit from the inner cleansing and will love the pure, clean feeling you receive! My father fasted religiously during his life as do I, and as do millions of our readers and students the world over, living The Bragg Healthy Lifestyle.

Purge Your Body of Toxic Poisons

The characteristics of tissue construction, especially of the important internal organs such as the liver, kidneys, lungs and glands, are all very much like those of a sponge. Now imagine a sponge soaked with a sticky glue or paste. As a person lives on the lifeless foods of civilization, the vital organs begin to fill up with this slimy paste or glue (*toxic poisons*). The vital organs actually become so clogged with decaying toxins that they can no longer function!

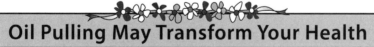

Oil Pulling May Transform Your Health

The ancient Ayurvedic remedy for oral health and detoxification is oil pulling! It involves the use of pure oil – as in organic olive oil or coconut oil, for pulling harmful bacteria, fungus and other organisms out of the mouth, teeth, gums and even throat. All you need to do is place about a tablespoon of oil into your mouth and swish it around for about 10-15 minutes, then please spit it out! Lipids in the oil pulls out toxins and the oil absorbs toxins and bacteria. The oil helps in cellular restructuring, proper functioning of lymph nodes and other internal organs. – *www.OilPulling.com*

I humbled my soul with fasting. – Psalms 69:10

We receive thousands of letters yearly from grateful students who have put our Bragg Healthy Lifestyle with fasting to the test and discovered it worked for them! Quite often, when every other method failed them, this Bragg Lifestyle proved successful! We want to inspire you, our reader and health friend, to improve your whole body, not just relieve a symptom! We are interested in your obtaining Super Health and Longevity! We love to hear your successes! Do write us!!

Fasting – Mother Nature's Master Healer

Mother Nature heals through FASTING every physical problem that's possible to heal! This alone proves that Mother Nature recognizes but one problem, that in every body the largest illness-causing factors are toxic poisons – decaying mucus, foreign matter, pus and uric acid. Just look at what happens to people when they suffer from a common cold. They run a high fever (body burning up toxins) while they eliminate great masses of mucus from the sinus cavities of the head, throat, lungs and bronchial tubes. A cold is the body's way of saying, *"I must rid the body of this toxic slime to survive!"* And a healing crisis is started by the body's Vital Force. Please reread this fasting chapter often to inspire you to fast to keep your body cleaner and healthier!

Fasting is a Safe, Effective Way to Detoxify the Body

"A technique wise men have used for centuries to heal the sick. Fast regularly and help the body heal itself and stay well. Give all of your organs a rest. Fasting can help reverse the ageing process, and if we use it correctly, we will live longer, happier lives. Just 3 days a month will do it. Each time you complete a fast, you will feel better. Your body will have a chance to heal and rebuild its immune system by regular fasting. You can fight off illness and the degenerative diseases so common in this chemically polluted environment we live in. When you feel a cold, illness or depression or allergy attack coming on – fast!"

– *James Balch, M.D., co-author, "Prescription for Nutritional Healing"*
Dr. Balch said, "Bragg Books were my conversion to Healthy Living."

Fasting helps remove mucus, toxins and obstructions,
arterial plaque and cleanses the entire body.

Fasting Cleanses, Renews and Rejuvenates

Our bodies have a natural self-cleansing and healing system for maintaining a healthy body and our "river of life" – our bloodstream. It's essential that we keep our entire bodily machinery from head to toes in perfect health and in good working order to maintain life! Fasting is the best detoxifying method. It's also the most effective and safest way to increase elimination of waste buildups while enhancing the body's miraculous self-repairing and self-healing process that keeps you healthy.

If you prepare for a fast by eating a cleansing diet for 1 to 2 days, this can greatly facilitate the healing process. Fresh variety salads, fresh organic vegetables and fruits and their juices, as well as green powder drinks, (choose from alfalfa, barley, chlorophyll, chlorella, spirulina and wheatgrass) stimulate waste elimination. Live, fresh foods and juices can literally pick up dead matter from your body and carry it away. Following this pre-cleansing diet, you can now start your detox water fast.

Daily, even during most fasts, we take 3,000 mg. of mixed vitamin C powder (acerola, bioflavonoids, rosehips and C concentrate) in liquids. This is a potent antioxidant and helps flush out deadly free radicals. It also promotes collagen production for new healthy tissues. Also vitamin C and grapeseed extract are both important if you are detoxifying from prescription drugs or alcohol overload.

A peaceful, well planned distilled water fast is our favorite. This fast can cleanse your body of excess mucus, old fecal matter, trapped cellular, non-food wastes and help remove inorganic mineral deposits and sludge from your pipes and joints. Fasting works by self-digestion. During a fast your body will perform cleansing miracles by intuitively decomposing and burning only the substances and tissues that are damaged, diseased or unneeded, such as abscesses, tumors, excess fat and excess water and the stored (stock piled) congestive wastes!

You are a Miracle – Self-Cleansing, Self-Repairing, Self-Healing –
Please become aware of "YOU" and be thankful for all your
miracle blessings that take place daily! – Paul C. Bragg, N.D., Ph.D.

Fasting Accelerates Elimination of Toxins

Even a relatively short fast (1 to 3 days) will accelerate elimination from your liver, kidneys, lungs, bloodstream and skin. Sometimes you will experience dramatic changes (cleansing and healing crises) as accumulated wastes are expelled. With your first fasts you may temporarily have headaches, fatigue, body odor, bad breath, coated tongue, mouth sores and even diarrhea as your body is cleaning house. Please be patient and loving with your miracle human home – your body!

After a fast your body continues to self-cleanse and healthfully rebalance! When you follow The Bragg Healthy Lifestyle, your weekly 24-hour fast removes toxins on a regular basis so they don't accumulate! Your energy levels will begin to rise – physically, psychologically and mentally. Your creativity will begin to expand. You will feel like a "different person" – which you are – you are being cleansed, purified and reborn. It's an exciting and wonderful miracle that is happening! Enjoy it!

Fasting Brings Remarkable Results

Professor A.E. Crews of Edinburgh University, who studied both worms and animals, stated: *"Given appropriate and essential conditions of the environment, including proper care of the body . . . Eternal Youth, in fact, can be a reality in living forms! It's been found to be possible by repeated processes of fasting, to keep a worm alive 20 times longer than it would have lived regularly. This has also been proven with animals."* Life-extending results have been proven again and again recently with an earthworm study. Something to think about, indeed, that proves the merits of fasting! Don't delay – start soon!

Remember, it took time for the body to build up toxins, so it takes time to cleanse and unload them! Take your time! Be faithful to The Bragg Healthy Lifestyle Program. You will reap wonderful, priceless benefits.

Fasting is an ancient natural healing practice that should be applied more today – it's safe, practical and very affordable.
– Michael Klaper, M.D., Hawaii

More Scientific Proof Fasting Works Miracles

Dr. Roy Walford, a famous University of California at Los Angeles Scientist and Life-Extension Researcher was a leading authority in dietary-restriction studies, with over 325 articles in scientific journals. He practiced dietary restrictions himself and never overate. He was the chief scientist of the Biosphere Study in Arizona. This experiment involved four men and four women living in a totally enclosed environment for one year. Their calories were restricted by 29%. During that time they all registered healthier, decreased levels in blood pressure, triglycerides, cholesterol and other toxins! These results were similar to studies conducted by Professor Crews of Edinburgh University on earthworms and animals.

Banish All of Your Fears About Fasting!

The average person has a preconceived notion that if they skip a few meals or fast for a few days, dangerous things will happen to their body. Nothing is further from the truth! My father and I have fasted for as many as 30 days straight – and felt stronger on the 30th day than when the fast started! Caution! We don't advise our students to go on long fasts unless needed and supervised by a health professional. *Please check with your health care professional before starting longer fasts.*

Nothing will give the body more energy and vitality than fasting. Fasting also strengthens the body's digestive system and immune system. Forget your fears! Fasting cleanses the internal body. Try a short fast to demonstrate to yourself the miracles fasting can accomplish in your life!

Fasting is your body's miracle "house cleaning" that focuses on removals, repairs and building of new cells! – Jason Fung, M.D.

Your body wants mucus and toxic slime out! Do all you can to help remove these toxins. When you feel them in your throat and sinuses, cough, spit and blow the mucus out. Your body works hard to collect these unwanted toxins. Please never swallow (recycle) mucus – get it out! Mucus and toxins are trouble-makers and a heavy burden when they stockpile. They can cause future disease and cancers! The main reason to live The Bragg Healthy Lifestyle (toxicless, mucusless) is that it promotes a healthy, clean body!

How to Conduct 3-Day, 7-Day & 10-Day Fasts

A fast of 3 days or longer should be conducted under ideal, peaceful conditions. You should be able to rest any time you feel the toxins passing out of your body. During this time you might feel some discomfort. You should rest and relax quietly until the poisons have passed out of your body. It's best to be quiet, at peace and alone when possible. This brief period of discomfort will end as soon as the loosened toxins have passed out of your body through the kidneys, liver, lungs and skin.

Our fasting is such a very personal and quiet time that many years ago Dad went into the beautiful Santa Monica Mountains in California and bought a tract of land in the wilderness of the Topanga Canyon near Malibu where he built a retreat cabin, similar to Thoreau's at Walden Pond near Boston. In that natural seclusion Dad and I enjoyed the quiet peace for our fasting time. If possible, try to get away to a secluded place to fast in solitude and Mother Nature's fresh air, to enjoy better results!

There are now very fine health spas worldwide where all the conditions are perfect for a restful fast. Inquire at health stores for any in your area. Many of our Bragg students who fast regularly tell us that they use their vacation as a period of fasting and purification of body, mind and soul. Some will rent a place in a quiet country setting to fast in seclusion. It's not necessary to go away from home to fast. Your home is your castle and hopefully you will be more at peace there. The Bragg family are all healthy fasters and, when one of us is fasting, we show consideration for each other. We have an agreement not to ask each other how we feel during the fast. Fasting is so personal that no one can do anything for you during the fast, so the best thing is not to discuss it with others.

When you are on a fast from 3 to 10 days or more, you are really on Mother Nature's miraculous cleansing operating table. Your body is purging the waste, mucus, toxins and other foreign substances out of your body that you had stored from unhealthy, wrong eating, etc.

Fasting cleanses, purifies and profoundly modifies our tissues.
– Dr. Alexis Carrel • NobelPrize.org

(BENEFITS FROM THE JOYS OF FASTING)

Fasting renews your faith in yourself, your strength and God's strength.
Fasting is easier than any diet.
Fasting is the quickest way to lose weight.
Fasting is adaptable to a busy life.
Fasting gives the body a physiological rest.
Fasting is used successfully in the treatment of many physical illnesses.
Fasting can yield weight losses of up to 10 pounds or more in the first week.
Fasting lowers and normalizes cholesterol, homocysteine, blood pressure levels.
Fasting improves dietary habits.
Fasting increases pleasure eating healthy foods.
Fasting is a calming experience, often relieving tension and insomnia.
Fasting frequently induces feelings of happy euphoria, a natural high.
Fasting is a miracle rejuvenator, helps in slowing the ageing process.
Fasting is a natural stimulant to rejuvenate the growth hormone levels.
Fasting is an energizer, not a debilitator.
Fasting aids the elimination process.
Fasting often results in a more vigorous happy marital relationship.
Fasting can eliminate smoking, drug and drinking addictions.
Fasting is a regulator, educating the body to consume food only as needed.
Fasting saves precious time spent on marketing, preparing and eating.
Fasting rids the body of toxins, giving it an internal shower and cleansing.
Fasting does not deprive the body of essential nutrients.
Fasting can be used to uncover the sources of food allergies.
Fasting is used effectively in schizophrenia and other mental illness treatment.
Fasting under proper supervision can be tolerated easily up to four weeks.
Fasting does not accumulate appetite; hunger pangs disappear in 1-2 days.
Fasting is routine for most of the animal kingdom.
Fasting has been a common practice since the beginning of man's existence.
Fasting is practiced in all religions; the Bible alone has 74 references to fasting.
Fasting under proper conditions is absolutely safe.
Fasting is a blessing – "Fasting As A Way Of Life" – Allan Cott, M.D.
Fasting is not starving, it's nature's cure that God has given us. – Patricia Bragg

137

Dear Health Friend,

This gentle reminder explains the great benefits from "The Miracle of Fasting" that you will enjoy when starting on your weekly 24-hour Bragg Fasting Program for Super Health! It's a precious time of body-mind-soul cleansing and renewal.

On fast days I drink 8-10 glasses of distilled (our favorite) or purified water, (I add 1-2 tsps. organic apple cider vinegar to three of them). If just starting, you may also try herbal teas or try diluted fresh juices with 1/3 distilled water. Every day, even on fast days, add 1 Tbsp. of psyllium husk powder to liquids once daily. It's an extra cleanser and helps normalize weight, cholesterol and blood pressure and helps promote healthy elimination. Fasting is the oldest, most effective healing method known to man. Fasting offers great miraculous blessings from Mother Nature and our Creator. It begins the self-cleansing of the inner-body workings so we can promote our own self-healing.

My father and I wrote the book "The Miracle of Fasting" to share with you the health miracles it can perform in your life. It's all so worthwhile to do. It's an important part of The Bragg Healthy Lifestyle.

With Love, *Patricia*

Paul Bragg's work on fasting and water is one of the great contributions to The Healing Wisdom and The Natural Health Movement in the world today.
– Gabriel Cousens, M.D., author "Conscious Eating" and "Spiritual Nutrition"

Blender/Juice Fast – Introduction to Water Fast

Fasting has been rediscovered, through juice fasting, as a simple, easy means of cleansing and restoring health and vitality. To fast (abstain from food) comes from the Old English word *fasten* or *to hold firm*. It's a means to commit oneself to the task of finding inner strength through body, mind and soul cleansing. Throughout history the world's greatest philosophers and sages – including Socrates, Plato, Buddha and Gandhi have enjoyed fasting and preached its many miracle benefits!

Although we feel a water fast is best, an introductory liquid juice fast can offer people an ideal opportunity to give their intestinal systems a restful, cleansing relief from the high fat, high sugar, high salt and high protein fast foods too many Americans unhealthfully exist on!

Organic, raw, live fruit and vegetable juices can be purchased fresh from Health Stores. You can also prepare these healthy drinks yourself using a good juicer/blender. When juice fasting, it's best to dilute juice with $1/3$ distilled water. The list on the next page gives many delicious combination ideas. With any vegetable and tomato combinations try adding some green powder (barley, chlorella, spirulina, etc.) to create a delicious, nutritious, powerful health drink. When using herbs in these drinks, use 1 to 2 fresh leaves or sea kelp – rich in protein, iodine and iron and delicious with vegetable juices.

Fasting is based on unchanging biological laws that insist the cause of disease must be removed. After hearing about a natural food diet and therapeutic, safe fasting, individuals may enthusiastically give it a try and get well! It is also possible they may become excited about the sensibleness of this approach and the prospect of finally recovering their health, but then go home to friends and family and become discouraged, after being told they would be crazy to attempt such an 'outrageous' treatment. They might even call a few uninformed doctors they know, only to be told fasting is risky and stupid.
– Joel Fuhrman, M.D., author of "Fasting and Eating for Health"

Following The Bragg Healthy Lifestyle and water fasting one day a week not only provides life extension, but an extra savings of 15% off your annual food bill. – Patricia Bragg

Paul C. Bragg Introduced Juicing to America

Juicing has come a long way since the first hand operated vegetable-fruit juicers from Europe were available. Before, this juice was pressed by hand using cheesecloth. He introduced his new juice therapy idea, then pineapple juice, then later tomato juice, to the American public. These two juices were erroneously thought to be too acidic. Now, these health beverages have become the favorites of millions. TV's famous *Juicemen* Jay Kordich and Jack LaLanne say Paul Bragg was their early inspiration and mentor! LaLanne also has a great juicer. They both loved living The Bragg Healthy Lifestyle and inspiring millions to health.

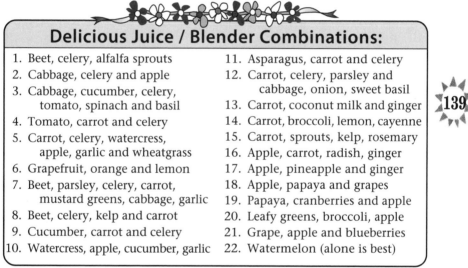

Delicious Juice / Blender Combinations:

1. Beet, celery, alfalfa sprouts
2. Cabbage, celery and apple
3. Cabbage, cucumber, celery, tomato, spinach and basil
4. Tomato, carrot and celery
5. Carrot, celery, watercress, apple, garlic and wheatgrass
6. Grapefruit, orange and lemon
7. Beet, parsley, celery, carrot, mustard greens, cabbage, garlic
8. Beet, celery, kelp and carrot
9. Cucumber, carrot and celery
10. Watercress, apple, cucumber, garlic
11. Asparagus, carrot and celery
12. Carrot, celery, parsley and cabbage, onion, sweet basil
13. Carrot, coconut milk and ginger
14. Carrot, broccoli, lemon, cayenne
15. Carrot, sprouts, kelp, rosemary
16. Apple, carrot, radish, ginger
17. Apple, pineapple and ginger
18. Apple, papaya and grapes
19. Papaya, cranberries and apple
20. Leafy greens, broccoli, apple
21. Grape, apple and blueberries
22. Watermelon (alone is best)

139

Liquefy or Juice Fresh Organic Fruits & Veggies

The juicer, food processor and blender are great for preparing foods, drinks, gentle (bland) diets and baby foods. Fibers of juiced fresh fruits and vegetables can be tolerated on most gentle diets. Any raw or cooked fruit or vegetable can be liquefied and added to broth, soups and non-dairy (rice or nut) milks. Fresh juices supercharge your energy level and boost your immune system to maximize your body's health power. You may fortify liquid meals or Bragg Smoothies with any green vegetable powders, alfalfa, barley green, chlorella, spirulina and wheat grass for extra nutrition.

Banish Constipation Mother Nature's Way

Constipation is often referred to as the cause of many serious physical health problems. Yet few people know what a normal bowel movement means. The average person feels that if they have one bowel movement a day they are not constipated. This is not true! People who only have one daily bowel movement are chronically constipated and carry 5 to 10 pounds of putrefying, fermenting food material in their lower bowel. This produces irritation to the delicate lining of the bowel. The bowel then either tries to get rid of the irritations quickly – which results in diarrhea – or puts a spastic clamp on the intestines to keep them from producing further – resulting in constipation and other health problems.

Civilized people never seem to go to the root cause of their constipation – an unhealthy lifestyle, lack of sufficient water (8-10 glasses of distilled or purified water daily is a must), no exercise and weak internal and external muscles of the abdomen. Americans spend over a billion dollars yearly trying to move their constipated bowels. In fact, all of the civilized countries sell large amounts of laxatives to move their cemented bowels.

The chief reason Americans need so much bowel "dynamite" is because they eat so much refined, mushy, lifeless, unnatural and empty-calorie food. The refined grains and other foods have lost the B-complex vitamins needed to have a healthy and clean intestinal tract (see page 143). Their digestive tract will lack tone unless vitamin B1 is present. Most diets consist of too many over-cooked, mushy, junk and fast foods that lack the tough cellulose fibers of raw vegetables that act as helpful, tiny intestinal brooms to give mobility, bulk, moisture and lubrication to the colon.

Organic whole grains, vegetables, fruits, raw nuts and seeds give needed vitamins and minerals to the body. – Patricia Bragg

Increasing intake of fruits and vegetables can help you prevent cancer and other chronic diseases. Surveys show those who increased their daily fruit and vegetable intake improved their health, vitality and well-being.
– UC Berkeley Wellness Letter • www.BerkeleyWellness.com

Raw Fresh Vegetables and Fruits Promote Healthy Elimination

The Bragg Healthy Lifestyle emphasizes at all times that a person should have 1 to 2 raw coarse salads a day. The base of these salads should be raw chopped or grated cabbage, carrots, beets, and celery. (See page 72 for our famous Bragg Healthy Salad Recipe!) The fleshy part of raw vegetables and fruits, contain cellulose, a colloidal element that retains water and acts as a soft bulk throughout the entire digestive system and helps promote health and good elimination! If for some reason you can't eat coarser raw foods, you can grate or blend them – or if you simply can't tolerate them – then grind 2 Tbsps flaxseeds (great over veggies, soups, etc.) or make a flaxseed tea (page 143) and drink 20 minutes after meals.

8-10 Glasses Distilled Water Daily Promotes Super Health and Also Healthy Elimination!

141

Cleanliness of the colon is important for superior health. See that your daily liquid intake is at least 8 glasses of distilled or purified water, plus some vegetable or fruit juices, especially if bowel movements are dry. If you are troubled by rectum soreness or hemorrhoids, try a peeled garlic bud – oiled with olive oil, inserted as a suppository and allowed to remain overnight. Aloe gel has also been found to be healing. Many people suffer from constipation due to dehydration because they don't drink enough water. Remember salt, black tea, coffee, alcohol, cola, soft drinks are dehydrating. One function of the lower bowel is to remove surplus water from the waste. If wastes are not evacuated or remain in the colon too long and a great deal of water is removed, then the stools become too hard to easily eliminate. This painful condition can even damage delicate colon membranes causing hemorrhoids.

Fruit bears the closest relation to light. The sun pours a continuous flood of light into the fruits, and they furnish the best potion of food a human being requires for the sustenance of mind, body and life.
– Louisa May Alcott, author "Little Women" 1868

There is nothing as important to your health as good bowel elimination! You should have a bowel movement soon after arising and one within an hour after each meal. Output must equal intake! Take care of this important function. Make it a practice to go to the toilet within 20-30 minutes after each meal. Don't say that you are too busy. Regular bowel elimination is vital to vigorous health. These poisons must be moved out of the body – no meal should stay in the human colon more than 36 hours. We have trained our bowels to move a meal out of our bodies in 16 to 18 hours, and never more than 24 hours. When the normal rhythm of bowel evacuation is reached, many of your physical problems will vanish!

For Easier Flowing Bowel Movements

It's natural to squat to have bowel movements. It opens up the anal area more directly. When on a toilet, putting feet up 6 to 8 inches on waste basket or footstool gives the same squatting effect. Now raise arms, stretch hands above head so the transverse colon can empty and roll out completely with ease. It's important for you to drink 8 to 10 glasses of pure water daily – it works miracles! After the dinner meal take 1 psyllium husk vegetarian capsule daily or do Flaxseed Tea Cleanse (see next page).

How to Improve Your Digestion

Millions have poor digestion which is aggravated by weak saliva-enzyme juices that causes: gas, heartburn and stomach bloating. Five minutes before mealtime, take 1 Tbsp. distilled water with $1/2$ tsp. raw, organic apple cider vinegar. Before swallowing, hold in mouth for a few seconds. This promotes saliva, which allows digestion to begin in the mouth. This small amount of diluted apple cider vinegar causes stomach digestive fluids to flow faster, better and the results are improved digestion!

ELIMINATE THE "DRIBBLES" EXERCISE:
To keep bladder and sphincter muscles tight and toned, urinate – stop – urinate – stop, four times, twice daily when voiding, especially after age 40. This simple exercise works wonders for both men and women!

Intestinal Health and B-Complex Vitamins

The muscles of the intestinal tract may become flabby and prolapsed if B-complex vitamins are not abundant in the diet. *(We take B complex tabs and extra subliminal B12 daily)*. These water-soluble vitamins are not stored, but are lost in perspiration and urine, so be sure to include in your diet foods rich in B vitamins. These foods include: raw wheat germ, blackstrap molasses, rice polishings, brown rice, barley, millet, quinoa, soybeans, lentils, dried peas and beans, cornmeal, buckwheat groats, mushrooms, broccoli, turnip and mustard greens, spinach, cabbage, peas, cantaloupe, grapefruit and oranges. It's also found in fish, beef steak, beef heart, lamb kidney and egg yolks – but we prefer the heart-healthy vegetarian sources!

Caution! Never, under any circumstances, use mineral oil as a laxative! It robs the body of the fat-soluble vitamins (A, D, E and K) that are waiting to be assimilated by the intestinal tract. Avoid all mineral oil products.

Colon hydrotherapy is a safe and effective way to heal constipation, digestive issues and improve overall health and vitality. The use of enemas is thousands of years old, and can gently cleanse your colon during a fast. Both colon hydrotherapy and enemas support the body in the important task of detoxification and cleansing.

FLAXSEED TEA CLEANSE: Mix 1 tsp. ground flaxseed in 8 oz. of water. Take three times per day. While helping to cleanse your colon, you will also benefit from the healthy nutrients flaxseeds contain. Or for hot tea you may boil 8 oz. water with 2 tsps. flaxseeds for 2-3 minutes. Let sit another three minutes, then strain while still hot and drink. Do this three times per day.

Do as I do – drink 3 apple cider vinegar drinks daily. 2 tsps of each apple cider vinegar and raw honey in an 8 oz. glass of distilled/purified water.
– Julian Whitaker, M.D., Editor of "Health & Healing Newsletter"

Natural vitamins, minerals and food supplements are good insurance factors in helping to keep the body well nourished, peaceful and healthy.

Avoid health-destroying habits:
sugar, fat, salt, refined foods and refined flours,
chemical preservatives, soda and alcohol.

Deadly Vaccinations – Don't Get Them!

Most people in the western world today think of vaccinations against infectious disease as great miracles of modern medicine. The sad truth is vaccines pose too many health risks. These days, children can get as many as 70 vaccines before they start first grade. There are about 200 more vaccines in the pipeline! Many doctors are now warning that there is a correlation between the rise in vaccines and growing incidence of asthma, allergies, cancer, chronic fatigue syndrome, attention deficit disorder, autism and many other ailments. Demand your rights to protect your children from compulsory vaccinations (some states permit religious or philosophical exemption). While all immunization laws have exceptions that you can use, the wording in each state differs, and you must know the exact wording for your state to make the proper request of waiver. You may call or write your state representative and ask for a copy of the immunization laws in your state. Making this available is part of his job, and it will be sent promptly.

144

Also, view *www.ThinkTwice.com* for more details on vaccine laws in your state. NOTE: It is recommended that you seek the advice of a qualified lawyer for accurate and updated information.

Learn more about this grave health risk, visit web: *www.nvic.org* and read this shocking informing book: *Vaccines: Are They Really Safe and Effective?* by Neil Z. Miller.

Toxic Silver (Mercury) Fillings

If you have silver fillings please consider having them removed carefully and safely. Replace with tooth colored, non-toxic composites. Minimize the exposures of mercury vapor, and be sure to find a "Mercury Safe" Dentist. Visit web: *DentalWellness4u.com* for more info.

UNHEALTHY GUMS CAUSE TOOTH LOSS: Here's help – millions lose their teeth due to unhealthy gums (pyorrhea) due to refined, sugary diets. The Bragg Healthy Lifestyle promotes healthy gums. Daily do ACV gargles (1 tsp. apple cider vinegar in half glass of water) and daily take CoQ10.

The greatest mistake you can make in life is to be continually fearing a mistake you might never make. – Elbert Hubbard, 1885

Chapter 12

Spiritual & Emotional Health Promotes Physical Health

Meditation and Prayer Build Inner Strength

It is in the peaceful silence of meditation and prayer that you find a higher power than yourself. This power can help, guide and direct you towards the healthy goals in life you are seeking.

It is important to set aside a period twice daily – morning and evening – during which time, the mind can go into meditation and prayer to build inner strength. There must be order and clear purpose to your thinking. Silently restate your new goals in life. Remember that you must displace the old, useless and damaging habits of thought with fine, bright, new healthy ideas.

Every constructive thought stimulates the nervous system with great vitality and vigor, and this sustained and powerful activity stimulates the entire body. Through meditation and prayer you are building a strong mind in a healthy strong body and you are opening that inexhaustible reservoir of energy and creative intelligence which lies within each human.

Meditation and prayer will help establish equilibrium in the mind, body and soul. It infuses you with new energy and expanded awareness, while it instills you with an inner calm and peace. You gain strength to do and to endure – to take the strains and pressures of life in stride.

I cannot overstate the importance of the habit of quiet meditation and prayer for more health of the body, mind and spirit.
"In quietness shall be your strength." – Isaiah 30:15

As a single footstep will not make a path on earth, so a single thought will not make a pathway in the mind. To make a deep physical path, we walk again and again. To make a deep spiritual path, we must think over and over the kind of thoughts we wish to dominate our lives. – Henry Thoreau

---

Open my eyes, to behold wondrous things out of Thy law. – Psalms 119:18

Simple Techniques of Meditation & Prayer

Meditation and prayer is powerful. It allows you to analyze your life in relation to your lifestyle, environment or with a particular person, thing, field of knowledge, principle, etc. In other words, you are getting yourself set for a glorious journey toward fulfilling your goals in life. You can proceed confidently knowing you have set yourself toward a destination or goal which you will achieve with lasting, rewarding success.

Everyone has the capacity for meditation and prayer and it can change and empower your life! The effects of daily meditation and prayer for whom you desire and want to be are blessings. Ask for it! You will notice benefits immediately.

True meditation and prayer are completely free from mysticism and hypnotism. It offers you the ability to adjust to the fast pace of living with increased energy, self-confidence and greater peace of mind. It gives glowing inner happiness and brings harmony to the mental, physical and spiritual faculties. In turn, your life gets fuller and stronger and becomes filled with daily miracles.

Daily meditation and prayer gives you the chance to strengthen your resolve to completely follow The Bragg Healthy Lifestyle. Your morning meditation and prayer allows you to plan your day constructively. Your evening meditation and prayer offers you the opportunity to review your day and evaluate your accomplishments and mistakes as you plan how to correct the latter. During meditation and prayer, the body experiences a state of peaceful repose more profound than sleep. Studies have shown that the pulse, respiration and metabolism slow down to levels below those ordinarily reached during sleep. People normally feel as refreshed following a session as they would after a nap.

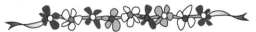

Count your blessings, name them one by one; count your many blessings, see what God hath done. – Johnson Oatman, Jr., songwriter
I give thanks for all the Miracle Blessings I receive daily. – Patricia Bragg

---

No man can violate Nature's Laws and escape her penalties! – Julian Johnson

Meditation and Prayer Helps Master Life

Taking inventory of yourself this way is important. You will soon notice a much greater peace, tranquility and health within yourself. Life will flow more easily for you. Annoying events, things and people that used to bother you will no longer have the same effect upon you. This will give you more energy for creative thinking and living.

The release, peace and relaxation that is experienced following meditation and prayer envelopes the entire day, with a softening effect upon your entire outlook and relations with life and others. The degree of personal involvement in emotional problems is diminished. This is not to say that emotional capacity is weakened! On the contrary, this wellspring is deepened as your inner life achieves greater life balance and stability. Meditation and prayer eliminates the causes of tension in a natural way (not like toxic tranquilizers), as it subtly sharpens the mind, heart and senses. This release from mental tension and physical duress creates a healthy effect on your entire well-being. Daily meditation and prayer helps to build a healthier balance to restore the body's normal rhythm of functions. Millions worldwide benefit from spirituality which gives practical and powerful guidance and love.

You Are What You Think and More

Turn your mind away from negative thoughts, but not in distaste and revulsion. Rather, turn eagerly toward that which is new, fresh and desirable – remembering the wisdom gleaned from past lessons. Look ahead to the many years you will have to enjoy what and who you are, because of the experiences you are living through today. Waste no energy on recriminations or self-pity, instead move forward toward the bright future with new energy!

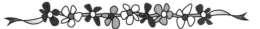

"A man is literally what he thinks. His character being the complete sum of all his thoughts." – Quote from "As a Man Thinketh" a literary essay by James Allen, published 1902

Please observe and respect the Laws of Mother Nature.

Control Your Negative & Positive Thoughts!

Think of your thoughts as powerful self-talk magnets with the ability to attract (positive) or repel (negative) according to the way used. A majority of people lean either to positive or negative mentalities. The positive phase is constructive and goes for success and positive achievements, while the negative side of life is destructive, leading to futility and failure. It is self-evident it is to our advantage to cultivate a positive, healthy, mental attitude. With patience, persistence and living The Bragg Healthy Lifestyle this can be accomplished!

Always keep in mind that whatever the mind tells the flesh, that is exactly what the flesh is going to believe and act upon. Your mind influences flesh.

Stress and Worry Eat Away at Your Health

148

Stress related diseases occur world-wide. In China, heart disease and stroke are projected to increase by 73% by the year 2030 or sooner! The country will lose $558 billion to these stress-related diseases, according to the World Health Organization. As in many parts of the world, decreased physical activity and unhealthy diets are leading to obesity, increased blood pressure and cholesterol and diabetes which ultimately leads to cardiac problems. (see web: *www.who.int*)

Most humans are so full of worry that they believe they can never overcome their miseries. Worrying about a problem does not solve it – it only makes things worse. As we said before, you can literally "worry yourself to death." A Hollywood neighbor of ours almost did!

> *Give me the Serenity to:*
> *Accept what cannot be changed;*
> *Courage to change what can be changed;*
> *and Wisdom to know the difference.*
> *- Reinhold Niebuhr*

Health and cheerfulness naturally beget each other. – Joseph Addison

---

If you truly love Nature, you will find Beauty everywhere.
– Vincent Van Gogh

Don't Worry, Please Be Happy & Healthy!

The good news is you can control all of these things in short time! Building positive attitude; maintaining a desire for lifelong learning and advancement; and most especially constantly working on reducing self-judgment and criticism, are all highly-effective at reducing stress. Daily try laughing out loud (*www.LaughterYoga.org*) and smiling at those around you. Learn to meditate or take relaxing walks; and make sure you assume responsibility for your life and what happens to you and don't blame others. This puts you in control, the Captain of your life, which helps immediately to reduce stress. Added to those efforts, of course, must be a healthy diet, regular exercise, and sufficient sleep. These are all valuable ingredients of The Bragg Healthy Lifestyle and once you make it part of your lifestyle, you will become stress-free, heart-healthy and live a longer, stronger, happier, fulfilled life.

To Over-Rest Mentally & Physically is To Rust

Remember your body will yield to your thoughts. You are what you think! By using your mind you sharpen its edge. Give it challenges with things to do and learn. Over-resting your mind gains nothing but its softening! Like the body, the more active you keep your mind, the better and sharper it will be. Recent studies show:

If you don't use it, you will lose it!

To over-rest mentally or physically is to rust. Get the negative thoughts out of your mind and demand more action from it! Let nothing and no one stop you in your quest for inner mental strength, peace and happiness!

As you follow The Bragg Healthy Lifestyle, you will feel the flow of new power surging throughout your entire body and soul. Summon into action your will-power and self-determination! Faithfully adhere to and work on your new positive thoughts daily. Remember, flesh is dumb. Make your body obey your mind!

To live is to know what counts and is important in your life. – Martin Grey

How Spiritual Beliefs Impact Healing

Spirituality shapes life's meaning for many people. Inside that meaning lies faith, which brings about trust, positive thinking and hope. Developing and nurturing spiritual values and a deeper sense of purpose can not only keep you healthy and well, but also provide the tools to grow, develop and heal when illness arises.

Numerous research studies are finding that those who have spiritual practices tend to live longer and that positive beliefs can influence health outcomes. Those who are spiritual tend to have a more positive outlook on life and a better quality of life. Spirituality helps people cope with disease and face the possibility of death with peace. By cultivating a spiritual life, people are able to gain strength, hope and the ability to counteract stress, which most experts believe is at the root of almost all diseases, illnesses and health conditions. Those with a spiritual perspective also tend to believe that disease and illness are the manifestation of negative emotions and thought patterns. Feelings like resentment, criticism, guilt and fear can all lead to an imbalance in the mind and body, creating physical illness that brings with it an opportunity for self-healing. Someone who takes a spiritual approach to illness will often heal once these negative deep-rooted beliefs are addressed and overcome.

Faith and Vision Create Miracles

When you begin to believe you can be what your inner vision tells you that you can become – that's when you're inspired. When you no longer see your weaknesses – but your strengths – then you discover the power and ability to do things you never dreamed of doing before!

During your daily meditation and prayer you must forget your inadequacies and reach inside to find your strength – it's there! See yourself as who you want to be. Paint a vivid picture in your mind. Concentrate on that image in your meditation and prayer times and carry it with you daily. By following The Bragg Healthy Lifestyle, you are working with Mother Nature, powers higher than yourself! You are then living by inspiration, one of the most tremendous forces in this great universe! Those happy, healthy, strong and vigorous people – those people who accomplish greatness – all those of faith, possess a deep spiritual philosophy. They believe that their lives are protected by a Power greater than their own. They believe there is a destiny which guides their lives. Nothing can thwart them! Following the Eternal Laws of Mother Nature they can accomplish great things!

Let Mother Nature Inspire You!

We'd like to urge you to ask Mother Nature to inspire you in your prayer and meditations and, while following our Healthy Lifestyle Program, to inspire you in your work, business and home. In Mother Nature you will find a power that will help you reach the heights of more healthy balanced living. Here are more great ingredients for a winning philosophy:

First: During prayer and meditations, dream great dreams and through meditation work to develop a will that translates those dreams into reality.

151

Second: Find inspiration in some great goal, some worthy cause or real challenge and let someone or something inspire you to see yourself not for what you are, but for what you can become and accomplish in life.

Third: Live by this Bragg Healthy Lifestyle Program, no matter what! Do the greatest good possible within you! Live up to the highest potential that you have! Accomplish those goals which have been set for you by Mother Nature! We know that if you meditate and pray twice to three times daily along these lines and build upon your inner strengths you will win, conquer and triumph with a long, happy, fruitful life!

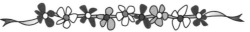

The real key to preventing heart disease is to use a combined approach, one that treats all facets of your physical and emotional health. It's extremely important to eat healthy real foods, get plenty of exercise, and address stress and your emotions, as too much stress and negative emotions will contribute significantly to heart disease. – DrMercola.com

Gloom and Bleakness steals joy, energy and color from your world. You can't save your life if you don't value it! – "Heart Healthy Living Magazine"

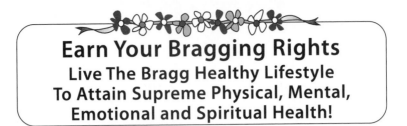

Earn Your Bragging Rights
Live The Bragg Healthy Lifestyle
To Attain Supreme Physical, Mental,
Emotional and Spiritual Health!

With your new awareness, understanding and sincere commitment of how to live The Bragg Healthy Lifestyle!

God bless you and your family and may He give you the strength, the courage and the patience to win your battle to re-enter the Healthy Garden of Eden while you are still living here on Earth with more years to enjoy it all!

With Blessings of Health, Peace, Joy and Love,

Paul and *Patricia*

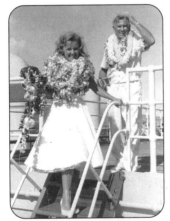

Health Crusaders Paul C. Bragg and daughter Patricia traveled the world spreading health, inspiring millions to renew and revitalize their health.

The Bragg books are written to inspire and guide you to health, fitness and longevity. Remember, the book you don't read won't help. So please reread Bragg Books and live The Bragg Healthy Lifestyle to enjoy a healthy fulfilled life!

I never suspected that I would have to learn how to live – that there were specific disciplines and ways of seeing the world that I had to master before I could awaken to a simple, healthy, happy, uncomplicated life.– Dan Millman, author "The Way of the Peaceful Warrior" • peacefulwarrior.com A Bragg fan and admirer since his Stanford University coaching days.

A truly good book teaches me better than to just read it, I must soon lay it down and commence living in its wisdom. What I began by reading, I must finish by acting! – Henry David Thoreau

Chapter 13

Questions & Answers About The Bragg Healthy Lifestyle

A Quick Look at Some Frequent Questions

We've traveled the world sharing The Bragg Healthy Lifestyle. We continually tell our health students as well as you, our readers and health friends, that our System is not a set of diets for specific ailments. The Bragg Healthy Lifestyle only recognizes one cause of human suffering and that is the clogging of the pipes and organs of the human body by toxic materials that have been deposited within its tissues due to an unhealthy lifestyle.

We are not in the curing business! We recognize no cures – except those that the body's internal, basic biological functions perform themselves! The body is self-cleansing, self-repairing and self-healing! Your body will do its best work when you do your best to give it a fair chance by following The Bragg Healthy Lifestyle.

153

Assist Mother Nature in this purification process and your physical problems will soon vanish. This System is not interested in the name of an ailment. We are only interested in what kind of wrong foods and beverages you have ingested and how long you have used them. If you have been saturating your tissues with toxic poisons for years, then you have built up large amounts of toxins which put pressure on your nerves and organs. This can cause aches, pains and worse, premature death!

When students ask us what they should do for a special ailment, we give but one answer, and that is to follow The Bragg Healthy Lifestyle and the water fasting to detoxify and cleanse. So many seem to think they should have a special diet for their special physical problem. That's not true. When the body is cleansed, it releases the toxic poisons and becomes purified – then there are no longer toxins to cause health problems!

He who has health has hope. He who has hope and God, has everything!

Most Frequently Asked Health Questions

Question: *I suffer from an inflamed colon. Raw fruits and raw vegetables give me gas pains when I eat them. How can I go on this diet, since I haven't eaten them in years? How can I eat them now?*

Answer: Of course you can't eat a lot of coarse raw fruits and vegetables at first! You will have to slowly start your program by using soft, mashed, cooked vegetables, stewed fruit such as apple sauce and then gradually add some soft, young, fresh lettuce.

Your one day a week water cure fast will help rest and heal your inflamed colon. No food will pass through your digestive tract for 24 hours. This gives your Vital Force a chance to do its healing work. It took you a long time to get into this condition! You must be patient and give your body a chance to heal this raw, inflamed digestive tract. Then have a day where you eat nothing but apple sauce or fresh vegetable juices. Also use Aloe gel (drink 1-2 Tbsps 3 times daily in juice or distilled water) and enjoy organic apple cider vinegar drink (recipe page 71) to help soothe/heal your digestive tract and colon.

Question: *Can a five-year-old child go on this program?*

Answer: Yes, in a modified way. A five-year-old child is growing and therefore must have the growth foods, such as soybeans, brown rice, beans, lentils and tofu, etc. Optional are some fertile eggs, goat's milk and natural cheese. Teach the child to enjoy raw and cooked vegetables, raw vegetable salads and fresh fruits along with nourishing growth foods (recipes page 72). A child of five should have 100% whole grain breads, cereals and pastas. Raw nuts and organic nut butters are perfect foods for growing children, as are raw wheat germ, spirulina and green barley powders.

Millions of Americans are committing slow suicide with their unhealthy, inactive lifestyle; heavy meat eating, sugar, salt and fat diets; plus smoking, drugs, and drinking alcohol. This all damages their organs and the inside of their arteries, adding graver health problems to their lives!
– Patricia Bragg, Pioneer Health Crusader

Question: *My children will not eat raw fruit, raw or lightly-cooked vegetables. All they want is junk, fast foods – meat, greasy french fried potatoes, hot dogs, hamburgers, white bread, pizzas, and sweets (candies, cakes, cookies, ice cream, sodas, etc). What should I do?*

Answer: You will have to take control of their health as a parent and guardian. Keep out of your home white refined breads, salty, fast junk foods, high fat, french fries, and deadly sugar candies and sweets, cola and soft drinks and diet aspartame drinks (page 64) and all foods listed on the "Foods to Avoid" list on page 19. There are wonderful cook books for healthy foods children love. Get your children in the kitchen, preparing foods with you! Let them choose which vegetables they would like to eat. Sweet baked yams and sweet potatoes are enticing tastes for children. Get creative! Offer them pastas made from lentils, chick peas, rice and quinoa. There are delicious healthy, sugar-free cereals available everywhere, as well as non-dairy milks. Smoothies are always a favorite!

We prefer you train them to enjoy healthier vegetarian meals! If you insist, occasionally they can have small portions of organically fed meat or fish with their salads and cooked veggies. But always have them eat a raw vegetable salad first before cooked foods.

It's your adult, mature mind overseeing your child's mind. You can slowly change meals over to healthy menus. Start to control the eating habits of your family! Remember, parents prepare with their two hands, food for their family – either Health or Sickness? It's up to you!

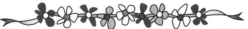

Children are very responsive to healthy lifestyle changes, and those start with providing the right foods (organic fruits, vegetables, whole grains and reasonable amounts of other healthy snacks) and encouraging regular hours for family meals, exercise, bedtime and wisely limit TV and web times. – Susan K. Rhodes, Ph.D., Medical University of South Carolina

*Researchers have discovered the more healthy habits an individual practices, the longer they live and the healthier and fitter they are!
– Elizabeth Vierck, author "Health Smart: Personal Plan to Living Longer"*

You are responsible for your family's health and well-being! Take charge, and be their caring, guiding Health Captain. – Patricia Bragg

Question: *Can a man who does hard physical labor live on The Bragg Healthy Lifestyle – The Toxicless Diet, Body Purification & Healing System and still keep up his strength?*

Answer: Eating heavy food does not produce physical strength. This is an old wives' tale that seems to live on. Many of our students do the hardest physical labor, yet they thrive on The Bragg Healthy Lifestyle. They have no heavy breakfast, only fruit. For lunch they may take several whole grain sandwiches and some raw nuts, seeds, vegetables and fruits, or a lunch of salads plus dried fruits and nuts. Some take a container of whole grain pasta or bean salad. We both have tested ourselves with hard physical labor and outside of eating a few more nuts and sunflower seeds – found we can work twelve hours and still feel peppy. It's a clean body that has strength and energy, not a body over-stuffed with heavy foods! We can climb high mountains even on only water or fresh fruits, trail-mix, nuts and dried fruits.

Question: *I don't seem to digest raw vegetables or fruits properly. Some pass out just as I ate them. Why?*

156

Answer: A weekly 24-hour fast and a periodic fast of three days will help restore the digestive juices to your digestive tract. We also recommend taking a digestive multi-enzyme with main meals. Also it works miracles to sip 1 Tbsp. distilled water with $1/2$ tsp raw organic apple cider vinegar before meals (see page 142). Your digestive system has been badly overworked for years. The coffee, sugar, starch, heavy meats and fats weakened it. Now it will take time to restore the digestive enzymes so you can handle these important health foods. Be patient – it takes time to rebuild the digestive system! Remember to chew each mouthful of food thoroughly! Your stomach has no teeth! This healthy habit improves digestion and health.

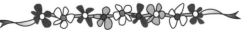

We know two things about how to prevent death in middle age: stop smoking and lower cholesterol. – Richard Peto, Oxford University

There is no trifling with nature; it is always true, dignified, and just; it is always in the right, and the faults and errors belong to us. Nature defies incompetence, but reveals its secrets to the competent, the truthful, and the pure. – Johann W. Goethe

Question: *Is it harmful to take a nap after a noon meal or to go to bed soon after your dinner meal?*

Answer: Children and babies, after eating, often take a nap. Most animals eat, then sleep. Your food digests whether you are asleep or awake. If you have your main meal during the day, and are able to rest afterwards, take a nap. We believe in naps when possible. This nap helps give you two days in one. You will awaken refreshed and ready for the rest of your day and evening. But, you must adjust to what is best for you and your time. In Europe and South America, short nap siestas after lunch are popular. Heavy lunches take your energy – avoid them, instead enjoy healthy salads, soups, veggies or fruits!

Question: *I have tried to fast for 24 hours, but I get so weak it's difficult to stay on my fast. I get headaches and feel sick in the stomach and some nausea. What should I do?*

Answer: This is a sign of detoxification. You may add vegetable juices to your fast, to give your body nutrients as you cleanse. You might consider colon hydrotherapy as well, to assist your body's release of toxins. Be patient! In time, your body will respond to the opportunity to fast by giving you energy and mental clarity. In the beginning, detox protocols such as colon hydro-therapy, enemas, salt baths and infrared saunas will relieve your detox symptoms.

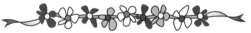

Your body is a non-stop living system, in constant motion 24 hours daily, cleaning, repairing, healing and growing. – Patricia Bragg

---

A full stomach doesn't like to think. – Old German Proverb

 The accumulation of toxins in the body accelerates ageing. The elimination of toxins awakens capacity for renewal. Toxins must be identified and eliminated from your body. Fasting is Mother Nature's cleansing miracle!

Wake up and say, "Today I am going to be happier, healthier and wiser in my daily living because I am the captain of my life and in control to steer it for 100% healthy lifestyle living!" Fact: Happy people look younger, live longer, are happier and have fewer health problems! – Patricia Bragg

---

Perfect health is above gold; a healthy body before riches. – Solomon

Question: *When I fast 24 hours – from dinner to dinner or breakfast to breakfast – time goes quickly. But on my 3 day fast may I have herbal teas to warm and console my stomach?*

Answer: Yes! Herbal teas like mint, alfalfa, chamomile, rose hip, dandelion, echinacea, goldenseal and anise, are soothing health beverages and are always permissible when you feel you need something warm in your stomach. If desired, you may add a small amount of raw honey, pure maple syrup or if diabetic try stevia herb drops to sweeten. Remember, most China black teas contain tannic acid, which is used to harden shoe leather, so from now on substitute herbal green teas (make sure they are decaffeinated!) You may also enjoy an apple cider vinegar drink (*recipe page 71*) several times a day (cold or hot) as it's a cleanser and purifier. Also, the juice of a fresh lemon in a glass of distilled water, sweetened with honey is permissible when fasting. Many feel this helps when fasting, while others prefer only distilled water. You decide.

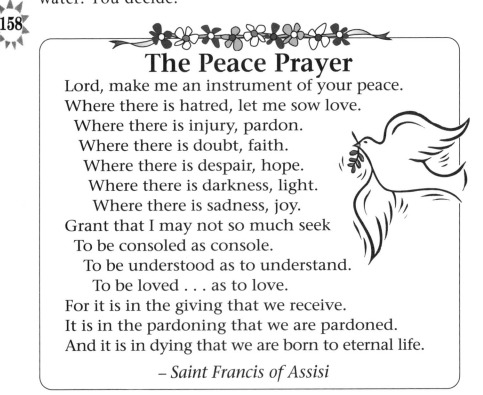

The Peace Prayer

Lord, make me an instrument of your peace.
Where there is hatred, let me sow love.
Where there is injury, pardon.
Where there is doubt, faith.
Where there is despair, hope.
Where there is darkness, light.
Where there is sadness, joy.
Grant that I may not so much seek
To be consoled as console.
To be understood as to understand.
To be loved . . . as to love.
For it is in the giving that we receive.
It is in the pardoning that we are pardoned.
And it is in dying that we are born to eternal life.

– Saint Francis of Assisi

Open your mind, for the doors of wisdom are never shut.
– Benjamin Franklin

Paul Bragg's South Seas Health Adventure

I had thoroughly enjoyed living on my Toxicless Diet, Body Purification and Healing System for many years with great results. Through the years I had progressively increased my intake of raw fruits and raw vegetables and lightly cooked vegetables. I had not eaten a regular breakfast for years.

I had fasted faithfully for one 24 to 36 hour period weekly for many years and had taken many, many cleansing fasts – some lasting from 7 to 10 days or longer. But now I was ready to go to the South Sea Islands and discover if it was possible to live on a 100% Toxicless Diet. I was seeking the Garden of Eden! I gave myself a year for the experiment. I sailed to Tahiti and based myself there. I also visited the smaller islands around Tahiti and I never stopped enjoying and living The Toxicless Diet, Body Purification and Healing System.

In Tahiti my diet was exclusively made up of raw tropical fruits and vegetables and lightly cooked vegetables. During this year I did not eat fish or flesh of any kind and no eggs, grains or any dairy products. I ate some raw nuts and seeds, especially when I took long trips – paddling the heavy outrigger canoe to the outer islands or while climbing mountains.

Daily, I exposed my body to the gentle early morning and late afternoon sun rays. I was often on lonely, deserted South Sea beaches where I could live at times absolutely nude. It was great!

With the healthy, pure, clean Toxicless Diet and the warm tropical sun, I became like one of the South Sea's Natives. In fact, when people did see me they would never believe I belonged to the Caucasian race! My skin and muscle tone were absolutely without a flaw. My strength, endurance, vitality, energy and vigor were supreme. Never before had I attained the physical and internal perfection that I reached on that great South Sea Adventure!

Good health, generated by physical fitness is the logical starting point for the pursuit of excellence in any field. Physical vitality promotes mental vitality and thus is essential to executive achievement.
– Dr. Richard E. Dutton, University of Southern Florida

Bragg Shares Found Secret to Total Health

Many people who have heard about my South Sea Adventure with The Toxicless Diet, Body Purification and Healing System have asked me, 'Why, if you attained physical perfection in Tahiti, did you leave that tropical Garden of Eden?' My only answer is that I had found the true secret to Total Health. I could not keep this life-changing health knowledge to myself! I knew I had to share my discovery with my fellow Americans and the world! I felt that now I had definitely proven that man can attain the highest state of physical perfection. I would have been selfish not to share it.

You can't be selfish and hold on to a great discovery! You must share and teach it. It's only by teaching that you, the teacher, come to know your subject better. I knew that I had been privileged to spend an entire year in the Garden of Eden. Knowing that few people could visit the South Seas like I did, I resolved to help others around the world to create their own Garden of Eden where they live!

Since I returned from my South Seas adventure, I have travelled around the world over 20 times. I've lived in all kinds of tropical, cold and temperate climates, but wherever I am I create my own Garden of Eden. In cold countries I add more natural starch to my diet, such as whole grain bread, pastas, natural brown rice, cereals and other products made from whole grains. I also use more raw nuts, seeds and nut butters. I may even add a few eggs or fish, but basically I don't care for flesh foods; I never did. I was reared on a big farm where I saw blood and slaughter at an early age, and it saddened me! There have been a few times when I ate meat and fish. I did research among the short-lived Eskimos in the Arctic Circle. If I had not eaten fish I would not be here today! I also studied the Laplanders, who live on reindeer meat. Again, without reindeer meat I would have starved. For most of my life I've enjoyed being a healthy vegetarian!!!

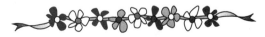

Roses are God's autograph of beauty, color and fragrance.
– Paul C. Bragg, N.D., Ph.D., Originator of Health Stores

Chapter 14

Healthy Alternative Therapies
and Massage Techniques

Try Them – They Are Working Miracles!

Explore these wonderful natural methods of healing your body. Finally over 600 Medical Schools in the U.S. are teaching Healthy Alternative Therapies. Please check their websites. Now seek and choose the best healing techniques for you:

ACUPUNCTURE / ACUPRESSURE: Acupuncture directs and rechannels body energy by inserting hair-thin needles (use only disposable needles) at specific points on the body. It's used for pain, backaches, migraines and general health and body dysfunctions. Used in Asia for centuries, acupuncture is safe, virtually painless and has no side effects! Acupressure is based on the same principles and uses finger pressure and massage rather than needles. Check web: *AcupunctureToday.com*

CHIROPRACTIC: was founded in Davenport, Iowa in 1885 by Daniel David Palmer. There are now many schools in the U.S., and graduates are joining Health Practitioners in all nations of the world to share healing techniques. Chiropractic is popular and the largest U.S. healing profession benefitting literally millions! Treatment involves soft tissue, spinal and body adjustment to free your nervous system of any interferences with normal body functions. Its concern is the functional integrity of the musculoskeletal system. In addition to manual methods, chiropractors use physical therapy modalities, exercise, health and nutritional guidance. Web: *ChiroWeb.com*

161

COLON HYDROTHERAPY: is a safe and effective practice for supporting detoxification, and improving health and vitality. Contact I-ACT (Int'l Association Colon Hydrotherapy) for a certified colon Hydro-Therapist in your area. Web: *i-act.org*

SKIN BRUSHING: daily is wonderful for circulation, toning, cleansing and healing. Use a dry vegetable brush (never nylon) and brush lightly. Helps purify lymph so it's able to detoxify your blood and tissues. Removes old skin cells, uric acid crystals and toxic wastes that come up through skin's pores. Use loofah sponge for variety in shower or tub.

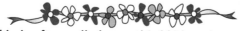

Skin is often called your third kidney because
it eliminates toxins from body.

Alternative Health Therapies & Massage Techniques

HOMEOPATHY: In 1796, Dr. Samuel Hahnemann, a German physician, developed homeopathy. Patients are treated with "micro" doses of remedies found in nature to trigger the body's own defenses. This homeopathic principle is a safe and nontoxic remedy and is the #1 alternative therapy in Europe and Britain because it is inexpensive, seldom has any side effects, and usually brings fast results. Web: *HomeopathyCenter.org*

NATUROPATHY: Brought to America by Dr. Benedict Lust, M.D., this treatment uses diet, herbs, homeopathy, fasting, exercise, hydrotherapy, manipulation and sunlight. Practitioners work with your body to restore health naturally. They reject surgery and drugs except as a last resort. Web: *www.Naturopathic.org*

OSTEOPATHY: The first School of Osteopathy was founded in 1892 by Dr. Andrew Taylor Still, M.D. There are now 30 U.S. colleges. Treatment involves soft tissue, spinal and body adjustments that free the nervous system from interferences that can cause illness. Healing by adjustment also includes good nutrition, physical therapies, proper breathing and good posture. Dr. Still's premise: if the body structure is altered or abnormal, then proper body function is altered and can cause pain and illness. Web: *www.AcademyofOsteopathy.org*

162

REFLEXOLOGY / ZONE THERAPY: Founded by Eunice Ingham, author of *Stories The Feet Can Tell*, inspired by a Bragg Health Crusade when she was 17. Reflexology helps the body and organs by removing crystalline deposits from reflex areas (nerve endings) of feet and hands through deep pressure massage. Primitive reflexology originated in China and Egypt and Native American Indians and Kenyans self-practiced it for centuries. Reflexology activates your body's flow of healing and energy by dislodging deposits. Visit Eunice Ingham and nephew Dwight Byer's website: *www.Reflexology-usa.net*

WATER THERAPY: Soothing detox shower: apply organic olive oil to skin, alternate hot and cold water, every 2-3 minutes. Massage body while under hot, filtered spray. Garden hose massage is great in summer or anytime. Hot detox soak bath (diabetics use warm water) 20 minutes with cup of Epsom salts or apple cider vinegar. This soak helps pull out the toxins by creating an artificial fever cleanse.

My father and I want you to enjoy a fulfilled, healthy, long life.
– Patricia Bragg, Pioneer Health Crusader

Time waits for no one, treasure and protect every moment you have!

ALEXANDER TECHNIQUE: helps end improper use of neuromuscular system, helps bring body posture into balance. Eliminates psycho-physical interferences, helps release long-held tension, and aids in re-establishing muscle tone. For more info see web: *AlexanderTechnique.com*

FELDENKRAIS METHOD: Dr. Moshe Feldenkrais founded this in the late 1940s. This Method leads to improved posture and helps create ease and more efficiency of body movement. This Method is a great stress removal. Web: *Feldenkrais.com*

REIKI: A Japanese form of massage that means "Universal Life Energy." Reiki Massage helps the body to detoxify, then re-balance and heal itself. Discovered in the ancient Sutra manuscripts by Dr. Mikao Usui in Japan 1922. Web: *Reiki.org*

ROLFING: Developed by Ida Rolf in the 1930's in the U.S. Rolfing is also called structural processing and postural release, or structural dynamics. It is based on the concept that distortions (accidents, injuries, falls, etc.) and the effects of gravity on the body cause upsets and long-term stress in the body. Rolfing helps to achieve balance and improved body posture. Methods involve the use of stretching, with gentle deep tissue massage and relaxation techniques to loosen old injuries, break bad movement and posture patterns. Web: *Rolf.org*

163

TRAGERING: Founded by Dr. Milton Trager M.D., who was inspired at age 18 by Paul C. Bragg to become a doctor. It is a mind-body learning method that involves gentle shaking and rocking, allowing the body to let go, releasing tensions and lengthening the muscles for more body peace and health. Tragering can do miracle healing where needed in the body frame, muscles and the entire body. Web: *Trager.com*

MASSAGE & AROMATHERAPY: works two ways: the essence (aroma) relaxes, as does healing massages. Essential oils are extracted from flowers, leaves, roots, seeds and barks. These are usually massaged into skin, inhaled or used in a bath to help the body relax, soothe and heal. The oils, used for centuries to treat numerous ailments, are revitalizing and energizing for the body and mind. Example: Tiger balm, MSM, echinacea and arnica help relieve muscle aches. (Avoid skin creams and lotions with mineral oil – it clogs the skin's pores.) Use these natural oils for the skin: almond, avocado, and I use organic olive oil and mix with aromatic essential oils: rosemary, lavender, rose, jasmine, sandalwood or lemon-balm, etc. – 6 oz. oil and 4 drops of an essential oil. Web: *www.Aromatherapy.com*

MASSAGE – SELF: Paul C. Bragg often said, *"You can be your own best massage therapist, even if you have only one good hand."* Near-miraculous health improvements have been achieved by victims of accidents or strokes in bringing life back to afflicted parts of their own bodies by self-massage and with vibrators. Treatments can be day or night, almost continual. Self-massage also helps achieve relaxation at day's end. Families and friends can learn and exchange massages; it's a wonderful sharing experience. Remember, babies love and thrive with daily massages, start from birth. Family pets also love soothing, healing touch of massages. Web: *RD.com/health/wellness/learn-the-art-of-self-massage*

MASSAGE – SHIATSU: Japanese massage form applies pressure from fingers, hands, elbows and even knees along the same points as acupuncture. Shiatsu originated in Japan and is based on traditional Chinese medicine, and has been widely practiced around the world since 1970s. Shiatsu has been used in Asia for centuries to relieve pain, common ills, muscle stress and to aid lymphatic circulation. See web: *centerpointmn.com/the-benefits-of-shiatsu-massage*

MASSAGE – SWEDISH: One of the oldest and the most popular and widely used massage techniques. This deep body massage soothes and promotes healthy circulation and is a great way to loosen and relax tight muscles before and after exercise. See web: *www.MassageDen.com/swedish-massage.shtml*

MASSAGE – SPORTS: An important health support system for professional and amateur athletes. Sports massage improves circulation and mobility to injured tissue, enables athletes to recover more rapidly from myofascial injury, reduces muscle soreness and chronic strain patterns. Soft tissues are freed of trigger points and adhesions, thus contributing to improvement of peak neuromuscular functioning and athletic performance.

Author's Comment: We have personally sampled many of these Alternative Therapies. It's estimated America's health care costs are over $2.6 trillion. It's more important than ever to be responsible for our own health! This includes seeking dedicated holistic health practitioners to keep us well by inspiring us to practice prevention! These Alternative Healing Therapies are also popular and getting results: aromatherapy, Ayurvedic, biofeedback, guided imagery, herbs, hyperbaric oxygen, music, meditation, magnets, saunas, tai chi, Qi gong, Pilates, Rebounder, yoga, etc. Explore them and be open to improving your earthly temple for a healthy, happier, longer life.

Seek and find the best for your body, mind and soul. – Patricia Bragg

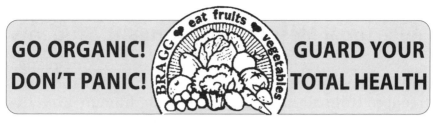

GO ORGANIC! DON'T PANIC! GUARD YOUR TOTAL HEALTH

FROM THE AUTHORS

This book was written for You! It can be your passport to a healthy, long, vital life. We in the Alternative Health Therapies join hands in one common objective – promoting a high standard of health for everyone. Healthy nutrition points the way – which is Mother Nature and God's Way. This book teaches you how to work with them, not against them! Health doctors, therapists nurses, teachers and caregivers are becoming more dedicated than ever before to keeping their patients healthy and fit. This book was written to emphasize the greatly needed importance of healthy lifestyle living for health and longevity, close to Mother Nature and God.

Statements in this book are scientific health findings, known facts of physiology and biological therapeutics. Paul C. Bragg practiced natural methods of living for over 80 years with highly beneficial results, knowing they were safe and of great value. His daughter Patricia lectured and co-authored Bragg Health Books with him and continues carrying on The Bragg Healthy Lifestlye.

165

Paul C. Bragg and daughter Patricia express their opinions solely as Public Health Educators and Health Crusaders. They offer no cure for disease. Only the body has the ability to cure a person. Experts may disagree with some of the statements made in this book. However, such statements are considered to be factual, based on the long-time experience of dedicated pioneer Health Crusaders Paul C. Bragg and Patricia Bragg. If you suspect you have a medical problem, please always seek qualified Health Care professionals to help you make the healthiest, wisest and best-informed choices!

Count your blessings daily while you do your 30 to 45 minute brisk walks and exercises with these affirmations – health! strength! youth! vitality! peace! laughter! humility! understanding! forgiveness! joy! and love for eternity! and soon all these qualities will come flooding and bouncing into your life. With blessings of super health, peace and love to you, our dear friends – our readers. – Patricia Bragg, Health Crusader

If I were to name the three most precious resources of life, I would say books, friends and nature; and the greatest of these, at least the most constant and always at hand is Mother Nature and God. – John Burroughs

A Personal Message to Our Health Students

It is our sincere desire that each one of our readers and students attain this precious super health and enjoy freedom from all nagging, tormenting human ailments.

After intelligent and careful study of this book, you now know that most human physical problems arise from a fermenting and decaying mass of toxins in the body. Many of these trouble spots are years old and are mainly concentrated in the intestines, colon and organs.

We have taught you there is no special diet for any one special ailment! The Bragg Healthy Lifestyle promotes cleansing through the eating of more organic raw fruits and vegetables combined with regular fasting. It's only through progressive cleansing that the human "cesspool" can be banished! We have told you you will go through healing crises from time to time. During these cleansing times you might have weakness and become discouraged! This is the time you must have great strength and faith! It's during these crises, when you feel the worst, you are doing the greatest amount of deep cleansing! You can create your own Garden of Eden anywhere you live, regardless of climate! All you have to do is purify the body of its toxic poisons by living a healthy lifestyle. You can reach a stage of health and youthfulness that you never thought possible!

You can feel ageless where your chronological age actually stands still and pathological age will make you younger! When your body is free of deadly toxic material you will reach a physical, mental, emotional and spiritual state that will give you happiness every waking hour as it adds many more youthful, active, joyous years to your life!

🌺 Bragg Healthy Lifestyle Plan 🌺

- *Read, plan, plot, and follow through for supreme health and longevity.*
- *Underline, highlight or dog-ear pages as you read important passages.*
- *Organizing your lifestyle helps you identify what's important in your life.*
- *Be faithful to your health goals everyday for a healthy, long, happy life.*
- *Where space allows we have included "words of wisdom" from great minds to motivate and inspire you. Please share your favorite sayings with us.*
- *Please write us on your successes following The Bragg Healthy Lifestyle.*

Index

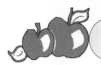

Index

B *(Continued)* . . .

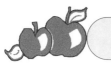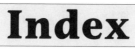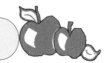

Index

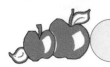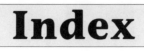# Index

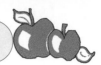

It's the song you sing and the smiles you wear,
that's making the sunshine everywhere. – James Whitcomb Riley

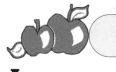

Index

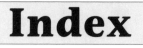

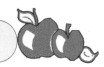

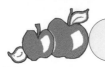 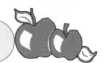

Index

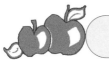

Index

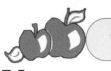

Index

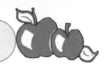

174

We are recharged and blessed by each one of you reading our
health books filled with loving health guidance for our readers
– thank you! – Patricia Bragg

Apple Cider Vinegar - Miracle Health System

BY PAUL C. BRAGG, N.D., PH.D.
and PATRICIA BRAGG

Paul C. Bragg, originator of health stores in America, and world-renowned health crusader Patricia Bragg, introduced America to the life-changing value of Apple Cider Vinegar, with the miracle enzyme known as "the mother." Now a widely popular beverage, this book reveals the legendary health-and life-giving versatility of apple cider vinegar. Following in the footsteps of Hippocrates, who taught the benefits of ACV to his patients in 400 BC, the Braggs teach dozens of reasons to use vinegar, including as a beauty aid, for skin treatments, in recipes, as an antibiotic, anti-septic, hair-revitalizing rinse, headache reliever, and weight reducer. ACV optimizes digestive health and can reduce or eliminate acid reflux. Paul and Patricia Bragg have helped millions heal and restore their vitality and zest for life through their time-tested understanding of natural health. *Apple Cider Vinegar: Miracle Health System* is informative, entertaining, and invaluable for anyone wanting to feel their best.

Bragg Healthy Lifestyle - Vital Living at Any Age

BY PAUL C. BRAGG, N.D., PH.D.
and PATRICIA BRAGG

Learn the simple strategies of radical health and vibrant wellness that The Bragg Healthy Lifestyle has brought to millions! What is an ageless body? For health pioneers Paul C. Bragg and Patricia Bragg, an ageless body sparkles with vitality, immune strength, mental clarity, and digestive ease. The Braggs teach why a toxic-free diet maximizes energy, supports weight loss, and can help heal illness and disease. In the newly revised *Bragg Healthy Lifestyle: Vital Living At Any Age*, the trailblazing father-daughter team who alerted us nearly a century ago to the dangers of sugar and toxic foods, detail every key aspect of creating and maintaining ageless health, including detoxification, stress-release, nutrition, exercise and the importance of taking charge of not only what goes into our bodies, but practices such as fasting, which release the toxins that may unnecessarily accelerate the aging process. "You are what you eat, drink, breathe, think, say and do," is the Bragg motto. From the foods we eat to our outlook, the environments we live in and even in our physical activities, the authors encourage readers to replace toxins with nutrients, flush out poisons and waste efficiently, exercise, breathe deeply and well, and cultivate happiness and harmony in our daily lives.

HEALTH SCIENCE
7127 Hollister Avenue, Suite 25A, Box 249, Santa Barbara, CA 93117
Toll-Free: (833) 408-1122

The Miracle of Fasting - Proven Throughout History

BY PAUL C. BRAGG, N.D., PH.D.
and PATRICIA BRAGG

In this newly revised best-seller, known to millions as the "bible of fasting" health pioneers and researchers Paul C. Bragg and Patricia Bragg teach why this ancient practice is key to health and energy, and critical to longevity and ageless vitality, due to our toxic environment and the stress of our daily lives. They share a detailed, step-by-step approach, accessible and informative for both beginners and experienced fasters. Our bodies must process not only our food and water, but the air we breathe, and whatever chemicals they may contain. Since detoxification and digestion take more energy than even strenuous athletic pursuits, fasting allows the mind and body to rest, renew and regenerate, to come into harmony and balance, and release the effects of stimulating foods like caffeine and sugars. The goal of fasting, say the authors, is to allow for the mind and body to self-heal. This concise, tightly edited *The Miracle of Fasting* is filled with personal stories of Paul C. Bragg's travels around the world, including a fasting journey in India with Mahatma Gandhi.

Healthy Heart - Learn the Facts

BY PAUL C. BRAGG, N.D., PH.D.
and PATRICIA BRAGG

Heart disease claims more American lives than any other illness and is the number one cause of death for women. World-renowned health pioneers Paul C. Bragg and Patricia Bragg teach time-tested, proven strategies for healing and maintaining a healthy heart for a long, active life! In a world filled with technological wizardry and products, the human heart still outperforms them all. That is – if that human heart is kept healthy. That is what the trailblazers Paul C. Bragg and Patricia Bragg have done in this book, sharing simple suggestions for lifestyle changes, nutritional support and exercises that will keep this most miraculous machine, your body, healthy and strong. You will learn how the heart works and how and why coronary disease is preventable and reversible. The authors provide an easy-to-follow blueprint for heart health that includes stress-release techniques, affirming that a positive mental outlook on life is a major element of heart health. The Braggs are legendary in the field of nutrition and health, and this newly revised and edited edition is a foundation of The Bragg Healthy Lifestyle. It is one of the most comprehensive heart health books on the market today.

Building Powerful Nerve Force & Positive Energy - Reduce Stress, Worry and Anger

BY PAUL C. BRAGG, N.D., PH.D.
and PATRICIA BRAGG

What is Nerve Force and why should you care about it? According to mental health trailblazers Paul C. Bragg and Patricia Bragg, "Nerve Force" is a type of life energy stored in the nerves, muscles, organs, and brain. The more Nerve Force you have, the quicker you can re-charge it, and the healthier, happier, and more satisfying a life you will lead. If you suffer from burnout, stress, fatigue, anxiety, insomnia or depression, this book is for you! We know that the ability to feel joy and peace is essential to a complete experience of vitality and wellness. Our thoughts, our attitudes, our outlook, and our emotional well-being are all dependent on having a powerful "Nerve Force." Just like any muscle that we can develop and strengthen, we can build our Nerve Force so that we are resilient, relaxed, and calm, even during times of stress. Paul C. Bragg and Patricia Bragg show you how with simple mental exercises and suggestions for specific foods that replenish your Nerve Force, as well as foods that deplete it, in this newly revised edition of *Building Powerful Nerve Force & Positive Energy* the father-daughter team explains to readers the reward of paying attention to the energy that is responsible for not only our physical capabilities and our vital body functions, but our ability to process information and feel centered and grounded, no matter what life throws at us. They teach us that maintaining a healthy Nerve Force, leads to a balanced and fruitful life.

Super Power Breathing - For Optimum Health & Healing

BY PAUL C. BRAGG, N.D., PH.D.
and PATRICIA BRAGG

Do you sometimes find that you are panting instead of breathing? Many of us do! This can cause headaches, anxiety, fatigue, and brain fog. The quality of our breath determines the quality of our life! This book teaches us how to breathe in a way that replenishes the body with the oxygen it so deeply craves. "The more effectively we breathe, the more effectively we live," write the authors, world-renowned health pioneers Paul C. Bragg and Patricia Bragg. "Super Power Breathing can make your life-force stronger, calmer and smarter." The Super Power Breathing program has been followed by Olympic athletes and millions of Bragg followers, and is filled with simple exercises for energizing and rejuvenating your breath, and your whole body. Research shows that we use only one-fourth to one-half of our lung capacity with each breath. This starves our body much like if we are depriving it of food. We are slowly robbing our body of its most vital, invisible nourishment – oxygen. In its newly revised form, the Bragg Super Power Breathing Program will give you all the tools you need to shift from shallow breathing to taking deep, oxygen-filled, life-giving breaths!

Water - The Shocking Truth

BY PAUL C. BRAGG, N.D., PH.D.
and PATRICIA BRAGG

The water you drink can literally make or break your health. The purity of our water is the most critical element in maintaining radical vitality, and healing from illness and disease. In this newly revised edition of *Water: The Shocking Truth*, health crusaders Paul C. Bragg and Patricia Bragg reveal the dangers of tap water, which research shows can be responsible for many ailments, due to the addition of dangerous chemicals such as fluoride and chlorine. In this book, the trailblazing father-daughter team teach the many functions water performs in the body, from regulating the various systems to flushing the body of waste and toxins. But what if the substance we use to cleanse our bodies is itself polluted? With the mandatory fluoridation of water in the municipal water systems, the authors assert that has been the case for decades. Added to the public water supply to prevent tooth decay starting in the 1950s, fluoride has long been known to be a toxin, used in pesticides and rat poisons. Learn what types of water are optimal to drink, how and why to detox your body with nature's most life-giving liquid, and the health-and-life-saving value of installing a water filter in your shower!

Bragg Back & Foot Fitness Program - Keys to a Pain-Free Back & Strong Healthy Feet

BY PAUL C. BRAGG, N.D., PH.D.
and PATRICIA BRAGG

If you are suffering with back or foot pain, look no further for a comprehensive program that will restore health to the parts of your body that carry you through life! Remember when we were children, and we had the kind of energy and flexibility to play for hours? Agile and active, we could twist, bend, stretch and climb with little effort. However, hours looking at a computer screen, a sedentary lifestyle and poor posture can take their toll. Eventually our backs start to hurt and cramp with every movement, and our feet ache after just a short walk. We start feeling "old." In *Bragg Back & Foot Fitness Program*, the father-daughter team of world-renowned health pioneers, Paul C. Bragg and Patricia Bragg teach how to speed the healing of injuries and develop a strong and flexible back and healthy feet, rejuvenating and re-energizing our bodies in the process. The trailblazing health experts who brought wellness and vitality to millions, including fitness guru Jack LaLanne, outline the keys to a healthy spine, pain-free back and bunion-free feet through nutritional support and clearly illustrated, simple exercises, as well as other tips for posture and massage. Paul and Patricia Bragg reveal the healing properties of herbs, effective ways to practice foot reflexology, how to deal with arthritis, athlete's foot, plantar fasciitis, and foot problems caused by diabetes.

By following the authors' Back and Foot Care Program, you can begin to treat your body as Mother Nature intended you to, and creating painless feet, a strong back and a powerful body will begin!

PATRICIA BRAGG
Health Crusader and "Angel of Health and Healing"

Author, Lecturer, Nutritionist, Health & Lifestyle Educator to World Leaders, Hollywood Stars, Singers, Athletes & Millions.

Patricia is a life-long health advocate and activist, admired internationally for her passionate work promoting healthy living. For many years she traveled the world, teaching The Bragg Healthy Lifestyle for physical, spiritual, emotional health and joy. She was invited to give lectures, visited radio shows, was profiled in magazines and appealed to people of all ages, nationalities and walks-of-life. Together with Paul, she co-authored a collection of ten books, with inspiration and techniques for living a long, vital, happy life. Now in her 90s and living on an organic farm in California, Patricia herself is a testament to these teachings and the sparkling symbol of health, perpetual youth and radiant energy.

PAUL C. BRAGG, N.D., Ph.D.
Life Extension Specialist • World Health Crusader
Lecturer and Advisor to Olympic Athletes, Royalty, Stars & Millions.
Originator of Health Food Stores & Founder of Health Movement Worldwide

Paul C. Bragg was at the forefront of the modern health movement, having inspired generations to turn toward wellness. At a young age, Paul turned his own health around by developing an eating, breathing and exercise program to build strength and vitality. From this life-changing experience, he pledged to dedicate the rest of his life to promoting a healthy lifestyle. He opened one of the country's first health food stores, which eventually led to the creation of the Bragg Live Foods company. With a devoted following, Paul traveled giving lectures and sharing his expertise, while serving as an advisor to athletes and movie stars alike. Even Jack LaLanne, the original television fitness guru, credited Paul with having introduced him to the importance of healthy living. In addition to the books Paul wrote with Patricia, they co-hosted television and radio shows and worked together to bring wellness to the world. Paul himself excelled in athletics, loved the ocean and the outdoors, and radiated with health and a warm smile.

Patricia inspires you to Renew, Rejuvenate and Revitalize your Life with "The Bragg Healthy Lifestyle" Books. Millions have benefitted from these life-changing philosophies with a longer, healthier, happier life!

Take Time for 12 Things

1. Take time to **Work** –
   it is the price of success.
2. Take time to **Think** –
   it is the source of power.
3. Take time to **Play** –
   it is the secret of youth.
4. Take time to **Read** –
   it is the foundation of knowledge.
5. Take time to **Worship** –
   it is the highway of reverence and
   washes the dust of earth from our eyes.
6. Take time to **Help and Enjoy Friends** –
   it is the source of happiness.
7. Take time to **Love and Share** –
   it is the one sacrament of life.
8. Take time to **Dream** –
   it hitches the soul to the stars.
9. Take time to **Laugh** –
   it is the singing that helps life's loads.
10. Take time for **Beauty** –
    it is everywhere in nature.
11. Take time for **Health** –
    it is the true wealth and treasure of life.
12. Take time to **Plan** –
    it is the secret of being able to have time
    for the first 11 things.

YOUR BIRTHRIGHT

HEALTH

CULTIVATE IT

Have an
Apple
Healthy Life!

3 John 2

*Teach me thy way, LORD, lead me in a straight path,
because of my oppressors. – Psalm 27:11*